BRADFORD W.G. PUBLIC LIBRARY

3 3328 00072952 1

D0856034

UE JUN 2 6 2006

DISCARDED

BRADFORD WG
PUBLIC LIBRARY

BRADFORD WG LIBRAR
100 HOLLAND COURT, BOX 13
BRADFORD, ONT. L3Z 2A7

WIN THE FAT WAR
for Moms

113 Real-Life Secrets to Losing Postpregnancy Pounds

CATHERINE CASSIDY
EDITOR-IN-CHIEF, *PREVENTION* MAGAZINE

MEDICAL CONSULTANT: SHARI BRASNER, M.D., *board-certified obstetrician and gynecologist*

RODALE

BRADFORD WG LIBRARY
100 HOLLAND COURT, BOX 130
BRADFORD, ONT. L3Z 2A7

Notice
This book is intended as a reference volume only, not as a medical manual. The information given here is designed to help you make informed decisions about your health. It is not intended as a substitute for any treatment that may have been prescribed by your doctor. If you suspect that you have a medical problem, we urge you to seek competent medical help.

© 2001 by Rodale Inc.
Cover photograph of Catherine Cassidy © by Hilmar
Profile photos courtesy of participants

All rights reserved. No part of this publication may be reproduced or transmitted in any form or by any means, electronic or mechanical, including photocopying, recording, or any other information storage and retrieval system, without the written permission of the publisher.

Prevention is a registered trademark of Rodale Inc.

Printed in the United States of America
Rodale Inc. makes every effort to use acid-free ∞, recycled paper ♻.

Cover Designer: Carol Angstadt
Series Cover Designer: Andrew Newman
Cover Photographers: Mitch Mandel/Rodale Images; Hilmar

Library of Congress Cataloging-in-Publication Data

Cassidy, Catherine, date.
    Win the fat war for moms : 113 real-life secrets to losing postpregnancy pounds / Catherine Cassidy ; medical consultant, Shari Brasner.
        p.   cm.
    Includes index.
    ISBN 1–57954–426–6   hardcover
    1. Postnatal care. 2. Weight loss. 3. Exercise for women. 4. Physical fitness for women.
    [DNLM: 1. Obesity—prevention & control—Popular Works. 2. Diet—Popular Works. 3. Exercise—Popular Works. 4. Puerperium—Popular Works. 5. Weight Loss—Popular Works. WD 212 C345w 2001] I. Brasner, Shari. II. Title.
RG801 .C37   2001
618.6—dc21
                                             2001000025

Distributed to the book trade by St. Martin's Press

2 4 6 8 10 9 7 5 3 1   hardcover

Visit us on the Web at www.preventionbookshelf.com, or call us toll-free at (800) 848-4735.

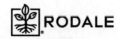

WE **INSPIRE** AND **ENABLE** PEOPLE TO IMPROVE
THEIR LIVES AND THE WORLD AROUND THEM

For all moms everywhere . . .
but especially for mine

Not too long ago, my friend and former colleague Anne Alexander wrote a wonderful little book called *Win the Fat War*. It became a bestseller. I'm grateful to Anne for recognizing the need for a book like hers. She laid the groundwork for *Win the Fat War for Moms*.

I also want to thank everyone on the *Prevention* Health Books team who contributed their time and talents to this project: Tammerly Booth, Susan Berg, Wyatt Myers, Elaine Czach, Leah Flickinger, Jennifer Bright, Deanna Portz, Beth Roehrig, Jennifer Goldsmith, Molly Brown, Teresa Yeykal, Carrie Havranek, Karen Neely, Darlene Schneck, Carol Angstadt, Bethany Bodder, Jodi Schaffer, Cindy Ratzlaff, Mary Lengle, Leslie Schneider, Dana Bacher, Lorraine Rodriguez, Tawan Smith, and Shannon Gallagher. Their dedication through months of hard work has been inspirational.

Special thanks, too, to my assistant, Carol Petrakovich. Without her dogged persistence, I would not have met my deadlines!

I also want to recognize Shari Brasner, M.D., a board-certified obstetrician and gynecologist and faculty member at Mount Sinai School of Medicine in New York City, for graciously sharing her time and expertise in shaping the book's content.

Of course, this book would not exist were it not for the 113 women who volunteered their stories to us. They answered the most personal of questions with grace and candor. To all of them, I offer my heartfelt respect and gratitude.

CONTENTS

INTRODUCTION

GOODBYE, BABY FAT!

When you're pregnant, everyone seems fascinated by your blossoming midsection. Total strangers ask you the sorts of questions you expect to hear only from your doctor—or your mother. And they're only too happy to shower you with advice: "*I* remember when I had *my* baby . . ."

Then you enter the ranks of motherhood, with a long-awaited bundle of joy—and some none-too-welcome postpregnancy pounds. Everyone else has lost interest in your midsection, but you can't stop worrying about it. Will the extra weight ever go away?

That's how I felt after I had my babies. That's why I jumped at the chance to do this book: I've been in your shoes, and I know how stubborn baby fat can be. But it *will* come off. It did for me.

With my first baby, I wasn't prepared for the weight gain. Actually, I wasn't prepared for pregnancy. I got used to the idea right about the time I began having problems. I was on complete bed rest, both in and out of the hospital, before giving birth to my son, Alex, in October 1989. He arrived via an emergency cesarean section, 3 months early. He died from complications just a month later, leaving me with a completely shattered heart.

By then I knew I wanted to have a family. But even when my doctor said I could try to conceive again, I needed time to grieve for Alex—and to lose about 12 postpregnancy pounds. I'd heard friends rave about Weight Watchers, so I signed up. I was diligent about keeping a food diary, exercising at the company gym, and going for my weekly weigh-ins. By March 1999, I was down to 111—5 pounds below my prepregnancy weight. (I'm about 5 feet 3, by the way.)

The following May, I became pregnant for a second time. I was determined to eat healthfully and exercise regularly. Then the cravings set in. I had a special fondness for red meat, eggs, chocolate-covered doughnuts, and anything from Taco Bell! I was taking a prenatal fitness class, which helped burn off the extra calories. But that came to an abrupt end in my sixth month, when I began experiencing cramping and contractions. My activity was restricted to walking—and even then, I had to be very careful.

All things considered, I was very lucky. I gained just 28 pounds before delivering my very healthy daughter, Jessica, in February 1991. Nursing my baby for 3½ months took off much of the weight. Still, I went back to work 12 pounds heavier. (It doesn't sound like much, but I'm a small person, and every pound makes a big differnce in the way my clothes fit.)

Once again I signed up for Weight Watchers—this time with a friend and colleague, Kerri, who'd just become a mom herself. We were the best of weight-loss buddies, going to our weekly weigh-ins together, taking walks at lunch and on weekends, splitting candy bars when our 3 o'clock chocolate cravings could not be ignored. I managed to get down to 115, and I was thrilled.

Staying at that weight wasn't easy. As my little girl got older and discovered ice cream, Oreos, and Kraft Macaroni and Cheese, I found myself eating foods I'd never before kept in the house. I also got in the habit of drinking a glass or two of wine in the evening, which didn't do my waistline any favors. And forget exercise: Between working full-time and raising a child, I had no desire to spend a minute of my "free time" working out.

Not surprisingly, I was up to 123 when I found out I was pregnant again. My fear of being even heavier afterward made me more conscientious about my eating habits and exercise routine. I curtailed my runs to Dunkin' Donuts and Taco Bell, though I did make some trips to Wendy's when Jess wanted "chickie nuggets" (I got a salad and baked potato). And I faithfully attended my prenatal fitness class through my sixth month, when contractions once again limited my activity.

Just about the same time, my doctor blindsided me with the news that I had gestational diabetes. I couldn't believe it. Why me? What was I doing wrong? What would happen to my baby? I went to a nutritionist, who calmed my fears and put me on a special diet—heavy on the fruits, veggies, and whole grains, light on the sugar. That was enough to clear up the diabetes within a month. As a bonus, it held my prenatal weight gain to 27 pounds.

My daughter, Jackie, arrived in October 1994—the Halloween surprise of a lifetime. She was a month early, delivered by cesarean section. Between childbirth and nursing, my weight dropped down to 126 rather quickly. And it stayed there.

You see, I had convinced myself that after three pregnancies, I could slim down on my own. But in reality, I wasn't eating all that well, and I just gave up on exercise. Even worse, my alcohol consumption was increasing in direct proportion to my stress level.

Finally, when Jackie turned 2, I went back to Weight Watchers. I also enrolled in a strength-training class at work. By May 1997, I was down to 117. I wanted to lose even more. I did, once I gave up drinking. After 6 months of abstinence, I reached 110—my weight when I graduated from college.

In the years since, I've managed to stay within 3 or 4 pounds of that weight. It's taken some work, that's for sure. But I've found a few tricks that seem to keep the scale right where I want it: I weigh myself regularly; I have breakfast—and a good lunch with lots of vegetables—every day; I don't eat after 9 o'clock at night; I stay away from alcohol; I get as much physical activity as I can, when I can (my favorite is ballroom dancing!); and I try to minimize stress, which unfortunately makes me eat.

This is what works for me. The women in the rest of the book have used a wide variety strategies to slim down after pregnancy. Each of us is unique in our bodies, our minds, and our circumstances. You need to identify the strategies that work for *you*. If you try something and it doesn't produce the results you want, don't give up. Just move on to something new. Through experience, you'll create a postpartum weight-loss plan that's tailored to you.

Where should you start? I suggest reading the three introductory chapters first. They provide general, expert-recommended guidelines for staying in shape during pregnancy (if you're still expecting) and for taking off the postpregnancy pounds (if you're already a mom).

The profiles themselves are organized into three chapters, for moms-to-be (Shape a Fit and Healthy Pregnancy), new moms (Lose the Postpartum Pouch), and moms who've had more than one baby (Win the War Once More). Of course, if you're pressed for time (and aren't most moms?), you may want to turn directly to the index. There you can look up profiles and strategies on specific topics, such as nutrition, exercise, and motivation.

The women you'll meet in this book are among the most remarkable human beings I've ever met. They're proof positive you can shed the baby fat and reclaim your figure after pregnancy. Be prepared to be amazed and inspired—and to blaze your own trail to weight-loss success!

Catherine Cassidy

—Catherine Cassidy
Editor-in-Chief, *Prevention* Magazine

The 10 Baby Steps
of Weight Loss

Congratulations—you're a mom! After 9 months of waiting and hoping, worrying and anticipating, you've been blessed with your very own bundle of joy. You couldn't feel more excited and proud.

Yet every time you look in the mirror, you wonder: "Now that the baby is here, will these extra pounds ever go away?"

Absolutely! In fact, you may be surprised at how quickly some of that baby fat disappears. Many moms say that losing the last 5 to 10 pounds—and keeping them off—is the biggest challenge. But it can be done. It just requires patience and perseverance.

To get you started down the path to postpartum weight-loss success, try adopting the following strategies. They're called the 10 Baby Steps of Weight Loss because each one moves you another step closer to your prepregnancy figure. Together, they form the foundation of an effective postpartum weight-loss plan.

What if you had your baby months ago and you're still trying to slim down? The Baby Steps can benefit you, too, providing direction and inspiration as you pursue your weight-loss goals.

Step 1: Enjoy Your Baby

As much as you may have prepared for your baby's arrival, your world is turned upside down anyway. Suddenly, you're responsible for not just one person but two. And as you've discovered, caring for a newborn is a 24-hour job. Needless to say, now is not the time to worry about weight loss. For the first 6 or so weeks after delivery, give your body a much-deserved rest. Use this time to get to know your baby; after all, the two of you have a lot of bonding to do.

While you don't want to launch a fat-burning workout just yet, with your doctor's approval you can do a few gentle exercises to stimulate your body's healing process. Kegels get the blood circulating to your most tender muscles again and can actually be done anytime following delivery. (For how-to instructions, see the chapter Yes, You *Can* Shed Those Pounds!) Some light stretching aids the recovery of your abdominal muscles as well as your back and legs. And if you can, walk at a leisurely pace for 15 minutes three times a week. Add 5 minutes per week if you aren't too tired. Walking is not only good exercise but also a great stress reliever for new moms.

When you look in the mirror those first few weeks, don't criticize yourself for carrying some extra pounds. Instead, celebrate your body for bringing a new life into this world—a wondrous, demanding, exhilarating achievement. You'll shed the baby fat soon enough. In general, women lose between 18 and 20 pounds within the first month after pregnancy.

Step 2: Set a Reasonable Goal

Once you've had your 6-week postpartum checkup and you've gotten your doctor's approval, you're ready to formulate your plan for slimming down and shaping up. Your first order of business is to establish your weight-loss goal. But you need to remember one important point: Your body has changed.

That's not to say you won't shed pounds. You will. But even then, some areas of your body, like your hips and thighs, may be a little more shapely than they were before you became pregnant.

At the 6-week mark, assess how many pounds you've lost naturally, without cutting calories or going full tilt on a fitness regimen. Use that as your baseline for deciding how much more you want to lose. Keep your goal small and measurable. If you're aiming to shed 20 pounds, consider dividing that into 5-pound increments. You'll feel that you're making progress, with each achievement inspiring you toward the next.

Once you decide on your goal, put it in writing. Post it where you'll see it constantly, like on the refrigerator or the bathroom mirror. Tell your family and friends about it, as long as they're supportive. You'll be less inclined to give up if you know that others are watching you.

Step 3: Establish a Schedule

You used to worry about your life becoming too predictable. Now you'd relish it! Ever since your baby arrived, your routine is far from routine. You may feel more time-crunched and exhausted than ever. And you may wonder whether you're ever going to get a chance to slim down.

Indeed, going off-schedule can open the door to some waist-widening habits. You may eat more prepackaged, processed food because you can't spare the time to cook healthy meals. And between getting up for early-morning feedings and being on the go all day long, you may not have the energy to even think about exercise.

Yet if you're committed to good nutrition and regular physical activity—the cornerstones of any successful weight-loss program—you *must* get yourself on a schedule. Just take your cues from your baby. Amid the feedings, the diaper changes, and the naps, you'll find opportunities to prepare a nutritious meal or to go for a short walk. Take advantage of them. As an alternative, perhaps your husband can watch the baby for an hour early in the morning or right after dinner, so you can go to the gym for a workout.

The point is, by reintroducing a little order into your life, you can free up some time for yourself. Then you can focus on your weight-loss efforts.

Step 4: Keep Stress in Check

Time, or a lack thereof, isn't the only challenge that new moms face. Sometimes the sheer responsibility of caring for a baby can become overwhelming. In fact, experts rank the birth of child among the most stressful of life events.

Your comfort with and confidence in your skills as a mom will undoubtedly grow with time. Right now, you need to take action to control your stress. If you don't, you may find yourself overeating, a common stress response that can lead to weight gain. It's just what you don't need when you're trying to lose baby fat.

What can you do to short-circuit stress? First and foremost, don't pressure yourself to be perfect. Allow yourself to make mistakes and to learn from them. Second, don't be afraid to ask for help. If family and friends offer to cook meals or run errands or watch the baby, accept their assistance without guilt. Third, find ways to squeeze in a little "quiet time": Meditate first thing in the morning; soak in a warm bath while your baby is napping; listen to relaxing music after dinner. Such brief respites can help you stay calm and in control the rest of the day. They can make all the difference in your fight against baby fat.

Step 5: Eat Smart, But Don't Diet

Eating nutritiously is just as important after pregnancy as during. Your body needs sustenance to support its recovery from the birthing process. And if you're nursing, your food choices have a direct effect on your baby.

Now is not the time to severely restrict calories. If you're significantly overweight, your doctor may advise you to make a moderate adjustment in your calorie intake. Even so, you should wait until you're nursing on a regular schedule (if you're planning to nurse) before changing your diet.

While you don't want to drastically cut calories, you can get them from the most nutritious sources. Plant foods—fruits, vegetables, beans, and whole grains—are always outstanding choices. They provide generous amounts of vitamins and minerals without a lot of fat. Meats and dairy products supply protein, along with other key nutrients. Just make sure they're lean or low-fat.

If you do opt to breastfeed your baby, you may actually need to *increase* your calorie consumption. That's because nursing typically burns around 500 calories per day. In fact, many of the women interviewed for this book say that nursing alone was enough to melt away their baby fat. In the first year after delivery, women who breastfeed tend to shed 4 to 5 pounds more than women who don't.

Nursing also stimulates the uterus to contract and shrink, which can initially help slim your abdomen and hips. Your body has many amazing ways of getting itself back into shape after pregnancy.

Step 6: Ease into Exercise

Pregnancy and childbirth demand a lot from your body. Your back, which has supported an enlarged uterus for several months, becomes sore. Your abdominal wall is stretched and sagging. Your pubococcygeus (PC) muscles, which have worked extra hard because of their location in the pelvic region, are exceptionally tender.

So once you get your doctor's approval to resume regular exercise—most likely at your 6-week postpartum checkup, depending on how quickly you heal—proceed *very slowly*. Your body needs to be treated gently, as it is still recovering from the birthing process. This is true even if you're a seasoned athlete.

Once you feel comfortable with light physical activity, you can gradually increase the intensity and duration of your workouts. Explore your options, and choose an activity that you enjoy. If you need a little extra motivation, consider signing up for an athletic event, like a charity walk/run. You may be more likely to stick with your training, and you'll feel a sense of accomplishment upon achieving your goal.

Step 7: Work Out with Baby

Can't exercise because of the baby? Then try including the baby in your fitness routine. Once your child has good head control (usually at 3 months, though you can check with your doctor to be sure), you can use a jogging stroller or a backpack-like child carrier to go walking. Your rhythmic pace might actually lull your little one to sleep. You can turn a set of crunches into a game of peekaboo. You can even lift your baby up and down for a little strength training.

Shaping up with your baby bestows many benefits. During the 30 to 60 minutes of your exercise session, the two of you can do lots of bonding. Your baby gives your workouts some strength-building resistance, while you expose your baby to an active lifestyle from a very early age.

Just remember that when you're exercising with an infant or toddler, you need to put the child's safety first. Provide adequate head and neck support at all times. Carry along fluids to prevent dehydration. To shield against the sun, cover your child's skin with clothing and a hat, or use a sun shield or canopy. While there's no danger associated with applying sunscreen, most pediatricians advise against exposing a baby's skin to sun at all.

Step 8: Maintain Your Motivation

Funny thing about motivation: You may not realize that you have it until it's gone. It can be especially tenuous for a mom who wants to slim down. You start out with the best of intentions, and your initial weight-loss success inspires you to pursue even loftier goals. But then the scale gets stuck, and you become distracted by the day-to-day demands of parenting. Just like that, your weight-loss efforts slip back to square one.

How do you rekindle your desire to slim down? To start, think about what you've accomplished so far. Maybe you've already lost a number of pounds. Maybe you've cleaned up your eating habits or established a regular fitness routine. The point is, you've made progress toward your goal. Do you really want to start over again?

Next, troubleshoot your existing weight-loss plan. If you've reached a plateau—you were getting thinner but haven't lost an ounce in weeks—you may need to trim a few calories from your eating plan (but no severe calorie restriction, unless advised by your doctor) or increase the intensity of your workouts. Burning more calories than you consume will melt away those extra pounds.

Once you jump-start your weight-loss efforts, look for ways to maintain your momentum. The women interviewed for this book have lots of creative suggestions, from buying a brand-new outfit in your prepregnancy size to hanging a postpartum photo on your refrigerator. Any of their strategies can inspire you to stay on track.

Step 9: Baby Yourself, Too

With your baby requiring so much attention, you may find that your own needs are getting short shrift. You deserve the same tender loving care that you're giving to your little one. After all, when you feel good about yourself, you have more confidence in your ability to achieve your weight-loss goals.

The best way to self-nurture is to do something for the sheer pleasure of it. It needn't be extravagant. You can take in a movie, sign up for a pottery workshop, or go to a day spa for an allover beauty treatment. Your options are limited only by your imagination.

Don't feel guilty about spending a few hours, or even a day or two, apart from your baby. You're doing both of you a favor by taking time to relax and rejuvenate. You'll feel better, physically and emotionally. And your baby will sense that.

What's more, a well-timed timeout from your usual routine gives you a fresh perspective on your weight-loss efforts. You're better able to focus on what you want to achieve and why. Your positive mindset can make all the difference between weight-loss success and failure.

Step 10: Let Nature Take Its Course

Perhaps a few months have passed since your baby arrived, and you're still carrying an extra 5 to 10 pounds. Try not to get frustrated. As mentioned earlier, the last few pounds of baby fat tend to be the hardest to lose. But just because they won't release their grip right now doesn't mean that they'll hang around forever.

The notion that women automatically become heavier once they've had babies is pure fiction, a myth that you're better off ignoring. Most new moms get to within a few pounds of their prepregnancy weight within 18 months of delivery.

So be patient. As long as you continue to eat healthfully and exercise regularly, those extra pounds are almost certain to disappear. You'll have the body you want before you know it.

Baby's Growing—
And So Are You

From the day you broke the news to your family and friends, you've heard the same comments over and over again—from your mom, your sister, your coworker, your neighbor. You've heard them so many times that you can predict who will repeat them next and when.

"You're eating for two now!"

"Stay off your feet. You don't want to overdo!"

And of course, people not only say these things, they actually expect you to *listen*. So at any social gathering that involves food, they'll be sure to send the extra helpings straight to your plate. And right after dinner, they'll pull you toward the recliner, imploring you to sit down and rest.

Their advice can make you feel good in the short run. But through 9 months of pregnancy, it can have unhealthy consequences for you and your baby.

As a mother-to-be, you really don't need to eat that much more

NUTRITION ADVICE FOR VEGETARIANS

If you're a vegetarian, you don't necessarily need to change your eating style once you become pregnant. You do need to make sure that you're getting adequate amounts of all of the important nutrients.

According to Andrew Weil, M.D., director of integrative medicine and clinical professor of medicine at the University of Arizona College of Medicine in Tucson, vegan moms-to-be are at greatest risk for running low on vitamin B_{12} and iron. Both nutrients come primarily from animal foods. Even if you don't eat dairy products or eggs, you can still get vitamin B_{12} from fortified products such as cereals, soy milk, and nutritional yeast. Similarly, whole grains, beans, and dried fruits are good sources of iron.

If you're concerned about not getting enough of these or any other nutrients, talk with your doctor about taking a multivitamin/mineral supplement.

than usual—on average, between 200 and 300 extra calories per day. If you go over that amount, especially if you're not exercising regularly, you may be stuck with some unwanted pounds after delivery.

What about prenatal exercise? Not so long ago, even the American College of Obstetricians and Gynecologists (ACOG) seemed against it, recommending just 15 minutes of physical activity at a time. But in 1994, ACOG updated its guidelines, realizing that moderate workouts not only help manage prenatal weight gain but also prepare the body for labor and childbirth.

So as much as those around you may insist otherwise, you can't abandon your healthy lifestyle just because you're expecting. It's more important now than ever. The only person you really need to listen to is your doctor. Work with him (or her) to establish a prenatal nutrition-and-fitness program that supports you and your baby. The following information, though not a substitute for professional medical care, can help ensure a healthy pregnancy—and a quick departure of those postpregnancy pounds.

The First Trimester: Prepare Yourself for the Long Haul

From the moment you became pregnant, your body has undergone a cascade of changes. It began producing more blood than usual, and to accommodate the extra volume, it increased your pulse rate by as much as 15 beats per minute. It also started using nutrients and water differently in order to nourish your baby.

During your first trimester, your doctor may advise you to start increasing your calorie intake. Remember, you only need 200 to 300 extra calories a day. Even though you're eating more, you may not gain any weight. That's okay. On average, moms-to-be gain only 2 to 4 pounds during the first 12 weeks of pregnancy. If you start losing weight, however, be sure to see your doctor.

To add calories to your diet, try to build your meals and snacks around low-fat, high-fiber, vitamin- and mineral-dense foods. You'll get the healthiest mix of nutrients by following the recommendations set forth in the USDA Food Guide Pyramid. The pyramid calls for at least nine servings of grains, four servings of vegetables, three servings of fruits, three servings of dairy, and three servings of protein. (For more information, see "Key Prenatal Nutrients and Their Sources" on page 12.)

Protein and calcium play key roles in a healthy pregnancy. Unfortunately, they usually come from high-fat foods like red meats and dairy products. Choose lean meats over well-marbled cuts, and low-fat or fat-free milk, cheese, and yogurt over full-fat varieties.

Even though you're consuming more calories, you don't want to waste them on nutritionally empty foods such as cookies, candy bars, potato chips, and pretzels. Sure, you can enjoy a treat once in a while. But overindulgence can lead to permanent postpregnancy pounds.

You might also want to keep an eye on your caffeine consump-

KEY PRENATAL NUTRIENTS AND THEIR SOURCES

Pregnancy alters your body's requirements for certain vitamins and minerals. This chart can safeguard against nutritional shortfalls that could prove harmful to you and your baby. The recommended intakes are specifically for moms-to-be, based on established government guidelines.

Nutrient	Recommended Daily Intake	Sources
Calcium	1,000 mg	Milk, cheese, and other dairy products; spinach; salmon and sardines; tofu; fortified juices and cereals
Folic acid	400 mcg	Green leafy vegetables, root vegetables, dark yellow fruits and vegetables, liver, salmon, broccoli, beans, nuts, milk, orange juice
Iron	30 mg	Lean red meats, shellfish, poultry, eggs, spinach, prune juice, dried fruits, whole grain breads and cereals
Magnesium	350 mg (ages 19–30); 360 mg (ages 31–50)	Green leafy vegetables, whole grains, fresh tuna, flounder, almonds

tion. Some experts recommend limiting yourself to 300 milligrams of caffeine a day, the amount in two 5-ounce cups of coffee or two 12-ounce glasses of cola. The caffeine may not contribute to prenatal weight gain, but the empty calories in soda sure will.

By eating well, you not only give your baby a healthy start, you also give yourself the best odds of slimming down soon after delivery.

Nutrient	Recommended Daily Intake	Sources
Vitamin A	8,000 IU	Spinach, mustard greens, carrots, sweet potatoes, cantaloupe, dairy products, eggs
Vitamin B_6	1.9 mg	Meats, bananas, whole grains, green leafy vegetables
Vitamin B_{12}	2.6 mcg	Milk, liver, meats, fish, poultry
Vitamin C	85 mg	Citrus fruits, tomatoes, broccoli, cantaloupe, green peppers, strawberries
Vitamin D	5 mcg	Dairy products, egg yolks
Vitamin E	15 mg	Vegetable oils, whole grains, nuts, seeds
Vitamin K	65 mcg	Spinach, cauliflower, eggs
Zinc	15 mg	Seafood, meats, peanuts, eggs, miso, pumpkin seeds

In the process, you just might minimize some of the physical discomforts that occur during pregnancy. Morning sickness is the classic example, affecting the majority of women during the first trimester, according to Lawrence Devoe, M.D., professor and chairperson of the department of obstetrics and gynecology and director of maternal-fetal medicine at the Medical College of Georgia in Augusta. You may also develop constipation, and you may have trouble sleeping. Certain

FOODS THAT FEND OFF PRENATAL DISCOMFORTS

During pregnancy, your body undergoes an enormous number of changes in order to accommodate and nourish your growing baby. Some of these changes may make you feel less than your best. But you may be able to get much-needed relief just by eating the right foods, as shown in the chart below from the Cleveland Clinic.

Symptom	Treatment
Abdominal pain	Get plenty of fluids.
Constipation	Eat lots of fresh fruits and vegetables. Drink at least eight 8-ounce glasses of water every day.
Diarrhea	Eat foods high in starch, such as breads, cereals, and rice.
Heartburn	Eat five or six small meals during the day, with a glass of milk before each. Chew your food slowly. Drink warm liquids, like herbal tea, but try to cut back on caffeine.
Leg cramps	Increase your intake of foods rich in calcium, such as milk, cheese, and fortified juices.

foods can help prevent and relieve these and other discomforts. (For more information, see "Foods That Fend Off Prenatal Discomforts.")

The Second Trimester: Now the Pounds Start Gaining On You

Women often refer to the second trimester as the golden period of pregnancy, and with good reason. The morning sickness finally sub-

Symptom	Treatment
Morning sickness	Have something dry—crackers, pretzels, or cereal—upon getting up in the morning, and a high-protein snack (such as lean meat) before going to bed at night. Eat five or six small, snack-size meals throughout the day, steering clear of fatty, greasy, and fried foods. Slowly sip fluids throughout the day.
Sleep problems	Drink a glass of warm milk at bedtime.
Stretch marks	Eat foods rich in vitamins C and E, nutrients that promote healthy skin.
Swelling in the extremities	Eat lots of high-protein foods, but avoid salty foods. Drink plenty of fluids.

sides, along with the sleep problems and persistent fatigue typical of the first 12 weeks of pregnancy.

Still, the physical changes come fast and furious. Consider this: By week 27, the end of your second trimester, your baby will have quadrupled in size.

This doesn't mean that you need to eat even more than you have been. As long as you're about 300 calories above your usual intake, and you're getting those calories from nutritious foods, you and your baby should be fine.

To ensure a consistent, healthy weight gain, you may want to consider dividing your standard three square meals a day into five or six small, snack-size meals. In addition, stock up on healthy snacks in case you need to feed a sudden attack of the munchies. Yogurt, dried fruit (including raisins), and peanut butter crackers are all good options.

The second trimester is prime time for another pregnancy phenomenon: cravings. Nearly two-thirds of all moms-to-be get them. The experts have yet to figure out why.

In Dr. Devoe's experience, most women seem to want foods at the extremes of the taste spectrum—things that are very sweet, very salty, or very bitter. "As long as these cravings don't take over your diet and prevent you from eating other, more nutritious foods, they shouldn't cause problems," he says.

Some women do develop cravings for substances that they normally wouldn't even eat—chalk, dirt, clay, or laundry starch, for example. This condition, called pica, is rare. But if it affects you, you absolutely need to see your doctor.

During your second trimester, your doctor may test you for gestational diabetes. About 4 percent of all moms-to-be develop this disease, which is usually diagnosed between the 24th and 28th weeks of pregnancy. While it has no well-defined outward symptoms, it's characterized by elevated blood sugar levels. Untreated, it can cause your baby to become too heavy or to develop breathing problems.

If you're found to have gestational diabetes, your doctor will likely instruct you to reduce your fat intake and eat more fresh fruits and vegetables—important strategies for any healthy pregnancy. The good news is, once you deliver your baby, your gestational diabetes will likely subside.

Be sure to seek prompt medical attention if you experience any sudden weight gain or loss at any time during your second trimester. From now until the end of your pregnancy, you should be putting on pounds at a slow but steady rate—just 1 to 2 per week.

The Third Trimester: Stay the Course until Baby's Arrival

As you approach your due date and your baby continues to grow, you're going to keep getting bigger . . . and bigger. You can expect to gain a total of 25 to 35 pounds before your delivery—more if you were underweight before your pregnancy, less if you were overweight.

During your third trimester, you may once again notice some physical discomforts. Many women experience shortness of breath, as the expanding uterus pushes the diaphragm (the muscle that lies beneath the lungs) out of place. Others report sleep problems, hip pain, hemorrhoids, and urine leakage. Virtually all of these discomforts result from continued weight gain. If any of them becomes particularly bothersome for you, ask your doctor what to do for relief.

Otherwise, just continue eating healthfully, as you have all through your pregnancy. You should be able to keep your prenatal weight within a healthy range. And once your baby is born, you should begin to shed most of those extra pounds.

WHEN YOU'RE EXPECTING MORE THAN ONE

Pregnancies with multiples—that is, more than one baby—have become quite common, largely because of an increase in the use of fertility drugs. In 1980, twins accounted for 1 in 56 births in the United States. But by 1996, that figure rose to 1 in 38.

While more babies bring more joy to the proud parents, they also create more responsibilities, especially during pregnancy. If you're carrying twins, for example, you need to increase your calorie intake by up to 450 per day. You can expect to gain between 35 and 45 pounds by the time your babies are born. This works out to about a pound a week during the first half of your pregnancy, and slightly more than a pound a week during the second half.

Research on other types of multiple births—triplets, quadruplets, and quintuplets, among others—is scant. Generally speaking, for each additional baby that you're carrying, you need to consume even more calories, and you can expect even greater prenatal weight gain. Your doctor can help you establish a nutrition plan that's tailored to your unique situation.

Exercise: Essential for a Healthy Pregnancy

With all of this talk about nutrition and eating, let's not lose sight of the other half of the prenatal fitness equation: exercise. The latest research has shown that moderate physical activity during pregnancy is not only safe, it's actually beneficial to both mom and baby.

In particular, women who engage in prenatal workouts experience fewer of the physical discomforts that often accompany pregnancy: swelling, leg cramps, shortness of breath, and fatigue. They're more successful at controlling their prenatal weight gain. And they recover quicker from the birthing process.

One study of recreational athletes who remained active through their pregnancies yielded some fascinating results. These women were far less likely than those who were inactive to require surgery to ensure a safe delivery. What's more, they had shorter labors (by 2 hours, on average), and their babies were subjected to less stress during the birthing process.

With your doctor's guidance, you should be able to establish some sort of prenatal fitness routine, no matter where you are in your pregnancy. If you've not been exercising regularly, your best bet is to choose an activity that won't jar your baby too much—something like walking, stationary cycling, or swimming. Yoga can be especially helpful, because it enhances bloodflow to the abdominal and lumbar (lower back) areas.

If you consider yourself a reasonably fit person and you have your doctor's approval, you may be able to push yourself a bit harder with activities such as jogging or low-impact aerobics. Still, some activities should be considered off-limits for the duration of your pregnancy, including contact sports and anything else that could endanger the baby.

Before You Move a Muscle . . .

While ACOG has relaxed its guidelines for moms-to-be, it still recommends moderate exercise, defined as any activity that has a woman working out at no more than 70 percent of her aerobic power. Rather than doing the calculations, your best bet is to work up to a heart rate of no more than 140 beats per minute, considered a safe and reasonable limit for most women during pregnancy.

Keep in mind that these guidelines are directed toward doctors, to help them safely prescribe exercise for their patients who are expecting. The recommendations do not apply to women with high-risk pregnancies. Before you undertake any prenatal fitness routine, talk with your doctor. He (or she) may want you to wear a heart monitor while you work out, so you can keep tabs on your level of exertion.

Once you're given the green light to exercise, the following strategies can help make your workout sessions safe.

- To avoid overheating your body, wear layers of clothes in light-weight fabrics (like cotton), so you can shed layers as necessary. Drink plenty of water, and keep your exercise environment cool.
- To protect your joints from injury, do 5 minutes of light physical activity before and after your workout.
- End your exercise session before full-blown fatigue sets in.
- During your second and third trimesters, avoid activities that have you lying on your back. It reduces bloodflow to your baby. For the same reason, try not to stand in the same position for too long.
- Because your sense of equilibrium changes as your baby grows, steer clear of movements that require good balance.

If you experience any of the following symptoms while you're exercising, stop what you're doing immediately and call your doctor.

- Contractions or abdominal cramping
- Dizziness or faintness
- Nausea
- Tingling sensations
- Swelling in the face, hands, or ankles
- Shortness of breath
- Stomach, back, or pubic pain
- Vaginal bleeding or water leakage

Armed with these guidelines and the advice of your doctor, you can stay active and fit throughout your pregnancy. That's good for you and your baby.

Yes, You *Can* Shed Those Pounds!

I n the African nation of Sudan, every new mom is treated like royalty. While her female relatives tend to her baby, she's free to relax and take care of herself for a full 40 days. Her only major responsibility is to breastfeed, and even then, her baby is delivered to her—no rolling out of bed for 2:00 A.M. feedings.

Why can't we have such a marvelous tradition? After all, as new moms ourselves, we certainly deserve some pampering for bringing a child into the world. Granted, we may get a little extra attention during the first week or two that we're home. And our spouses may help out whenever they can. But we assume the lion's share of the responsibility for the feedings, the diaper changes, and all of the other tasks involved in caring for a newborn.

Swept up in the whirlwind of motherhood, we can scarcely spare a moment to even think about taking care of ourselves. While setting aside your own needs in favor of your baby's is a noble gesture, in the long run, it isn't all that healthy. For one thing, you may feel so much stress that you eventually burn out and can't function as a caregiver. For another, you may settle into habits—like eating high-fat, high-calorie convenience foods or skipping workouts—that can keep you from shedding those post-pregnancy pounds.

Actually, you may feel better knowing that most of the extra weight goes away on its own. The majority of new moms get to within 5 pounds of their prepregnancy figures within 18 months of delivery, according to Eileen Behan, R.D., a nutrition consultant at Seacoast Family Practice in Exeter, New Hampshire. But those last 5 to 10 pounds can be the toughest to lose. And if you're not attending to your own body's needs—eating nutritious foods, including physical activity in your daily routine, taking well-timed "relaxation breaks"—the weight may start coming back.

Rest assured, you can reclaim your pre-baby body, whether you want to shed 5 pounds or 50. And you don't need to invest huge amounts of time or effort to succeed. In fact, just continuing your prenatal eating-and-exercise plan, with some modest adjustments, can help you slim down and shape up now that you're a mom.

Eating to Lose

Even though you've had your baby, you don't want to abandon the healthy eating habits that you established during your pregnancy. After all, your body has been through a lot, and it needs optimum nutritional support in order to fully recover from the stress of labor and delivery.

Of course, eating healthfully may seem more difficult now that a child has entered the picture. "Women are often motivated to eat well during pregnancy, but once the baby is born, they feel too stressed to pay attention to their own diets," explains Elizabeth M. Ward, R.D., a nutrition consultant based in Reading, Massachusetts, and a spokesperson for the American Dietetic Association. "They're at risk for shortchanging themselves nutritionally."

Feeding your body properly really isn't all that difficult. Just think plant foods—fruits, vegetables, beans, and whole grains. They deliver a range of key nutrients, but they tend to be low in calories and fat. That's important when you're trying to slim down.

What about meats and dairy products? They're excellent sources of protein, but they also tend to be high in fat. You can eat them, but choose low-fat or fat-free whenever possible.

While you want to be careful about your food choices, you don't want to significantly cut calories—at least not right after your baby is born. Remember, your body burns calories for energy. If you severely restrict your calorie intake, you may find yourself feeling absolutely run-down.

Breastfeeding? Good Nutrition Benefits Baby and You

For moms who opt to breastfeed their infants, adequate calorie consumption is especially important. In fact, they may need even more calories per day—up to 500 more—just to satisfy the energy demands of nursing.

This doesn't mean that you can indulge in a Big Mac or a banana split every day. Ideally, you should get those extra calories from nutrient-dense foods that support your baby's brain development. "Among the best choices are eggs, lean red meat, and fish such as canned salmon and fresh tuna," Ward says. "Eggs and lean red meat contain choline, a nutrient that fosters healthy neural development. And certain species of fish are rich in omega-3 fatty acids, another category of brain boosters."

Of course, if you do have an occasional Big Mac or banana split, you're probably not going to harm your baby. That's because the milk-producing cells in your breasts act as quality-control agents, regulating your milk's nutritional makeup. Essentially, they filter out the bad stuff before passing along the good stuff.

Still, certain foods that you'd ordinarily consider nutritious can produce adverse effects while you're nursing. For example, many mothers find that if they eat garlic, onions, broccoli, or cauliflower, their babies end up with gas, Behan says. Similarly, cow's milk has been linked with colic. If your baby seems to have a negative reac-

NECESSARY NUTRIENTS FOR NURSING MOMS

If you choose to breastfeed your child, you're going to need up to 500 extra calories a day. Try to get those calories from foods rich in the following nutrients, advises Judith Brown, Ph.D., coauthor of *Nutrition and Pregnancy: A Complete Guide from Preconception to Postdelivery*. All are important for mom and for baby.

Nutrient	Recommended Daily Intake	Sources
Calcium	1,000 mg	Milk, cheese, and other dairy products; spinach; salmon and sardines; tofu; fortified juices and cereals
Folic acid	500 mcg	Green leafy vegetables, root vegetables, dark yellow fruits and vegetables, liver, salmon, broccoli, beans, nuts, milk, orange juice
Iron	15 mg	Lean red meats, shellfish, poultry, eggs, spinach, prune juice, dried fruits, whole grain breads and cereals

tion after you've eaten a particular food, you may want to try eliminating it from your diet to see how your child responds.

While we're on the subject of adverse effects, you may be wondering what those extra 500 calories a day required for breastfeeding will do to your waistline. In all likelihood, they won't do anything. In fact, you can *lose* about ½ pound a week through nursing alone. As long as you don't lose too much too fast—no more than 2 pounds a month, or no more than 4 pounds a month if you were

Nutrient	Recommended Daily Intake	Sources
Magnesium	310 mg (ages 19–30); 320 mg (ages 31–50)	Green leafy vegetables, whole grains, fresh tuna, flounder, almonds
Vitamin A	6,500 IU	Spinach, mustard greens, carrots, sweet potatoes, cantaloupe, dairy products, eggs
Vitamin B_6	2 mg	Meats, bananas, whole grains, green leafy vegetables
Vitamin B_{12}	2.8 mcg	Milk, liver, meats, fish, poultry
Vitamin C	120 mg	Citrus fruits, tomatoes, broccoli, cantaloupe, green peppers, strawberries
Vitamin D	5 mcg	Dairy products, egg yolks
Vitamin E	19 mg	Vegetable oils, whole grains, nuts, seeds
Vitamin K	65 mcg	Spinach, cauliflower, eggs
Zinc	19 mg	Seafood, meats, peanuts, eggs, miso, pumpkin seeds

overweight before you became pregnant—you shouldn't notice any changes in your milk production.

If you're not breastfeeding, you may worry that you're more likely to retain your postpregnancy pounds. Don't. You can still trim and tone your postpartum body. Because you're not burning calories through nursing, you'll need to use them up some other way. For you, exercise may be the answer.

Exercise: A Must for Healing— And Weight Loss, Too

The key to postpartum exercise is to ease into it gradually. After all, your body has already endured a lot—9 months of pregnancy, plus hours of labor and the actual delivery. As much as you want to get rid of that baby fat, you're just not ready to go all out in your workouts. Your body needs time to rest and recuperate. With a baby to tend to, you don't want to end up battling fatigue.

In the first few weeks after giving birth, you can work on strengthening and toning your pubococcygeus (PC) muscles—the ones that work hardest during pregnancy and childbirth—by performing Kegels. These exercises are very easy to do, once you get the hang of them.

To start, you need to identify your PC muscles, which line your pelvic floor. The next time you urinate, try stopping the flow of urine in midstream. You're squeezing your PC muscles. Remember this sensation, so you can be sure that you're doing your Kegels correctly.

What's nice about Kegels is that you can practice them just about anywhere. Try to hold each one for 3 seconds, and repeat as often as you can. You may not be able to do too many at first, since your PC muscles are so tender. Gradually work up to 50 to 100 a day.

Beyond Kegels, you may benefit from some light stretching,

like pelvic tilts to strengthen your abdominal muscles (see the instructions on page 272) and shoulder shrugs to minimize strain in your lower back. Walking is another wonderful postpartum activity. It lays the groundwork for what will hopefully become a regular fitness routine. And it gets you out in the fresh air and sunshine—an effective antidote for frazzled nerves.

If you have any questions about which physical activities you can do, and when you can do them, talk with your doctor. Every woman recovers from pregnancy and childbirth at her own unique pace. While you certainly want to establish some sort of postpartum exercise program, you just as certainly don't want to push yourself too hard too soon after delivery.

Go Slow, But Get Moving

As a general rule, you should be ready to resume your regular fitness routine about 6 weeks after your baby's arrival. You'll likely be scheduled for a postpartum checkup at about that time. Ask your doctor whether you can add a bit more oomph to your exercise. Remember, the greater the intensity and/or duration of your workouts, the more calories you burn, and the more pounds you lose.

Once you have your doctor's approval, you can gradually increase your activity level. The operative word is *gradually*. Start with two or three 15- to 20-minute workouts a week, each at a moderate intensity. Your goal is to advance to three to five 30- to 60-minute workouts, each at a slightly higher intensity, over the course of a month.

If you were in good shape before your pregnancy, you may be able to progress at a faster pace. Just be careful not to overdo. Your body still needs time to get back in the swing of a regular fitness routine, especially if you cut back on your workouts while you were expecting.

What's the best postpartum physical activity? Anything that

works the body parts most affected by pregnancy, especially your abs, back, hips, and thighs. These areas can benefit from walking, cycling, swimming, and low-impact aerobics, as well as strength training.

Of course, for many new moms, the main concern about postpartum exercise is not what to do but when to do it. You can always ask your spouse or another family member to watch the baby while you work out. Or you can find a reputable gym that offers child-care services to its members. Don't feel guilty about leaving your baby for such a short time. You need the break, physically and emotionally.

If you can't bear to leave baby behind, you can always include him (or her) in your fitness routine. Buy a "sling" or a backpack-like child carrier, so you can take your baby on long walks. A jogging stroller would also work well once your baby has good head and neck control, usually after 3 months. The extra weight adds some muscle-building resistance to your workout. And some women say that the smooth motion of walking actually lulls their children to sleep.

You can even use your baby as a tiny "barbell," lying on your back and lifting him (or her) overhead. Again, just be sure that your baby has good head and neck control and is well-supported while you're working out. Excessive bouncing can lead to serious injury.

One other factor to consider: If you're nursing, try to schedule your workouts after your baby's feedings. You'll feel much more comfortable exercising when your breasts are empty than when they're full.

Situations Requiring Special Postpartum Care

As mentioned earlier, most women are able to get back into a regular fitness routine about 6 weeks after delivery. This rule does have some exceptions, however. If you've had a cesarean section or an episiotomy, for example, you may need to move a bit more slowly in your pursuit of a slimmer figure. "In these cases, I usually recommend waiting 10 to 12 weeks, even for women who've already had their 6-week postpartum checkups," says Michelle Mottola, Ph.D., associate professor of anatomy and kinesiology at the University of Western Ontario in London and director of the university's exercise and pregnancy laboratory. "They can still walk, but they should lay off the abdominal exercises until they feel better."

In fact, all of the following situations require extended recovery periods. If any of them apply to you, you need to exercise some extra care and caution when you're launching (or relaunching) a fitness routine.

If you've had a cesarean section: The first few weeks after a C-section are crucial. Your abdominal muscles are very tender, and you don't want to do anything to strain them. Still, some gentle exercises can support healing and recovery. The ones described on page 30 can even be practiced in bed, in case your doctor has instructed you to rest.

If you've had an episiotomy: An episiotomy is an incision made between the vagina and rectum to increase the size of the birth canal during labor. The incision needs time to heal. Kegel exercises can increase bloodflow to the area, which stimulates the healing process. They may feel uncomfortable at first, but they do help.

If you have diastasis recti: In some moms-to-be, the two halves of the abdominal muscles split down the middle to make room for the growing baby. If this happens to you, you may notice a bulge where the two muscles have separated. This phenomenon, called diastasis recti, prevented your muscles from tearing during your pregnancy. But now it needs to be watched carefully. If the gap is three finger-widths or greater (your doctor can help you measure), you need to avoid demanding abdominal exercises. Once the gap

CESAREAN-SAFE EXERCISES

If you delivered your baby by cesarean section, your physical activity may be restricted for a few weeks longer than usual so that your abdominal muscles can mend themselves. But this doesn't mean that you can't do anything at all. In fact, according to Shari Brasner, M.D., a board-certified obstetrician and gynecologist and faculty member at Mount Sinai School of Medicine in New York City, you can start the following exercises the week after your baby is born. They'll tone your abdominal muscles and support the healing process.

Abdominal breathing. Lie on your back with your knees bent. Cross your hands above your navel. Breathe deeply, inhaling for 5 seconds and exhaling for 5 seconds. You should feel your stomach rise with each inhalation. Repeat four to six times.

Pelvic tilts. Lie on your back with your knees bent. Exhale slowly. Tilt your pelvis upward as you flatten the small of your back. Inhale slowly, tightening your abdominal and buttock muscles. Then exhale slowly as you release your muscles. Repeat four to six times.

Leg slides. Lie on your back with your knees bent. Repeat the pelvic tilt exercise, only as you exhale the second time, straighten one leg while keeping the other bent. Inhale as you return the straight leg to a bent position. Repeat five times with each leg.

Ankle circles. Lie on your back with your knees bent. Raise one leg and rotate your ankle first in one direction, then the other. Repeat with the other leg, making sure to do 10 to 15 complete rotations with each ankle.

shrinks to two finger-widths, you can increase the intensity of your abdominal workout. Be sure to support your muscles by splinting, which involves crossing your hands over your lower abdomen to hold the muscles' seam in place.

If you've had a multiple birth: "You can easily include one baby in your fitness routine," Dr. Mottola says. "Two or three babies, or more, are a greater challenge." As soon as your doctor says you can exercise—remember, you may need more than 6 weeks to recuperate from childbirth—you should make arrangements for someone to watch your little ones while you work out. You need to get out of the house, if only for 15 to 20 minutes. "Caring for that many infants at once can be totally overwhelming," Dr. Mottola observes. "If you can step out for a while, you'll come back feeling relaxed and refreshed."

If you've had more than one child: You may have noticed that your recovery time has slowed down after each delivery. That's not because of the number of pregnancies. More likely, it's because of age. Quite simply, as you get older, healing takes longer. You may need a little more than the usual 6 weeks to get back on your feet. Beyond that, the guidelines for resuming a fitness routine are pretty much the same, whether you've had one child or four.

Shape a Fit and Healthy Pregnancy

SHE PLANNED FOR HER BABY FAT

After a year of trying to conceive, Susan Eugster was almost ready to see a fertility specialist. Then in July 1999, one last pregnancy test came out positive. "I was totally psyched," says the 33-year-old book designer from Emmaus, Pennsylvania. "I had finally gotten pregnant, and I was determined to do it right."

Susan's top priority was to stay healthy, for herself and her baby. That meant keeping her prenatal weight gain under control. "My mother told me about the adage that women shouldn't gain more than 20 pounds while they're pregnant," she explains. "My mom is pretty trim, and all of my siblings were born healthy."

With her doctor's okay, Susan plotted out how much she could gain each month to end up with no more than 20 extra pounds on her 5-foot-4½, 120-pound frame. But she promised herself that she wouldn't panic if she went over her goal. "My doctor told me that anywhere from 25 to 35 pounds was considered healthy, so I wasn't obsessing," she says. "I wasn't stepping on the scale every day."

Next, Susan shifted her attention to her eating and exercise habits—the two keys to managing prenatal weight gain. An avid runner, she intended to continue her workouts until her baby was born. But she had to abandon that plan under doctor's orders, after she experienced spotty bleeding early in her first trimester.

As disappointed as she was to give up running, Susan didn't worry about packing on the pregnancy pounds. "I just focused even more on eating well," she says. At breakfast, she'd eat yogurt, some fresh fruit, and a glass of orange juice. For lunch, she'd have a vegetable-laden salad, another piece of fruit, and a pint of low-fat milk. "Dinners weren't so balanced, because I didn't have time to cook," she says. "I ate my share of pizza and Mexican takeout. But I completely gave up soda and alcohol, drinking plenty of water instead."

Once into her second trimester, Susan got her doctor's okay to resume her running regimen. She put in 3 miles three or four times a week all the way into her ninth month. "Running not only made me fit, it kept my stress level down and my energy up," she says.

By the time she delivered daughter Gretchen in February 2000—after a lightning-quick 2-hour labor—Susan had gained 27 pounds, just 7 more than her goal. She had no trouble losing the baby fat, thanks to smart eating, regular exercise, and breastfeeding.

Within a week of the delivery, Susan was wearing her prepregnancy jeans. "They were tight," she says. But they gave her hope. Today, she weighs 9 pounds less than before she got pregnant.

WINNING ACTION

Set a weight-gain goal at the start of your pregnancy. *You'll be better able to manage your prenatal weight if you know up-front how much you can healthfully gain. Your doctor can help you establish an appropriate goal. Just be flexible about it. As long as you're eating well and exercising regularly (with your doctor's okay), your body will take care of the rest. Susan is proof of that! (She appears with her daughter on the cover.)*

SHE MADE UP HER MIND TO BREAK THE MOM MOLD

Even before she became pregnant for the first time, Alexis Davis didn't buy into the notion that welcoming a baby meant saying goodbye to a shapely physique. She firmly believed that moms could look sensational, too. Judging by her own postpartum weight-loss success, she was right!

Alexis has always been very conscientious about her weight. "I wouldn't describe myself as naturally slim," says the 35-year-old Plymouth, Indiana, resident. "I've had to work hard at it. Maybe that's why I was so attuned to pregnancy weight gain."

When she looked around at moms her age, Alexis noticed that many of them struggled with their postpregnancy pounds. They had a soft, round appearance—what Alexis describes as the stereotypical mommy look. "Some women get comfortable with it. But not me," she says. "I wanted people to look at me and say, 'Wow! You've had kids?'"

From the outset of her first pregnancy—with daughter Allegra, now 3½ years old—Alexis made every effort to control her prenatal weight gain. "I was already an avid exerciser, so I had a head start on staying fit," she says. "And as the chef/owner of a restaurant and catering company, I knew how to prepare foods in ways that would be very low in fat."

Indeed, running a business had Alexis maintaining a schedule that would bring most people to their knees. "I was on the go from 7:30 in the morning until 11:30 at night," she says. "My doctor told me that if I didn't take off the last week before my due date, he'd put me in the hospital. I did shorten my hours, heading home at 5:00 instead of 11:30, but just for 3 days. My baby arrived early!"

By the time she gave birth to Allegra, Alexis had added 36 pounds to her 5-foot-4, 119-pound frame. She returned to her job just 10 days after delivery; 2 months after, she began working out on a treadmill. That and eating healthfully were enough to melt away the leftover pounds in just 4 months.

Having proven to herself that she could regain her prepregnancy figure, Alexis cut herself a little slack during her second pregnancy a little more than 2 years later. She didn't work such long hours, though she made sure to stay active. She continued to eat well, too, using her culinary talents to whip up tasty, nutritious meals for herself and her family.

Even with her more lenient lifestyle, Alexis managed to limit her prenatal weight gain to 36 pounds, just as in her first pregnancy. She lost all of the weight within 6 months of delivering daughter Giuliana, now 16 months old.

These days, Alexis is even slimmer than before she became a mom, weighing in at 116 pounds. "I work only part-time, so I can be home with my daughters," she says. "But they really keep me on my toes! As long as I'm running after them, I won't need to worry about that baby fat coming back."

W I N N I N G   A C T I O N

Think positive from the start of your pregnancy. *Moms don't "automatically" get heavier once they've had their children. So don't just resign yourself to a fuller figure. Know that you can slim down after your baby arrives—and that a healthy prenatal lifestyle can set the stage for speedy postpartum weight loss. That's not all: By taking care of yourself now, through good nutrition and regular exercise, you're giving your baby the best possible chance of a healthy start in life.*

COUNTING CALORIES KEPT THIS MOM ON HER TOES

As a ballerina with the Milwaukee Ballet Company, 25-year-old Karisa Mae Stich Skiba had lots of motivation to get back into shape after the birth of her first child, Joshua, in May 2000. Just 6 months later, she would be dancing in the company's production of *Don Quixote*—in front of 2,200 people!

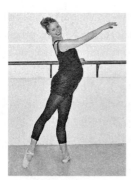

5 months pregnant

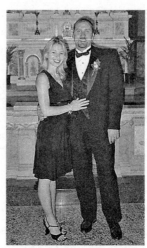

2 months after delivery

Karisa's strategy was simple and sensible. "I knew that if I could maintain a healthy weight gain during my pregnancy, I wouldn't have much to lose afterward," she explains. Daily ballet classes, plus aerobic and strength-training workouts several times a week, provided plenty of exercise. As for her eating habits, "I concentrated on making every calorie count toward having a healthy baby," she says.

Karisa certainly faced her share of temptation from sweets like cookies and cheesecake. But she adopted a practical technique to control her cravings. Just as many people rely on budgets to manage their personal finances, Karisa developed a budget to manage her calorie intake. Based on advice she had been given during previous visits to nutritionists, she determined how many calories she could consume per day, then planned how she would use them. This taught her to "spend" her calories wisely, on fruits and vegetables rather than fries and pizza.

With her doctor's approval, Karisa continued dancing all the way through her eighth month, even performing onstage during her second trimester. "Joshua was in the spotlight before he was even born," she muses. By the time her son made his official debut in the delivery room, Karisa had added 31 pounds to her 5-foot-5, 118-pound body. She was back to 124 just 6 weeks later, at her postpartum checkup. "I lost the last 6 pounds once I resumed my ballet classes and workouts," she says.

Karisa is thrilled that her body is gradually returning to dancing form. "I'm very critical of myself," she admits. "I work so hard to stay lean and muscular that I worried about becoming soft and flabby during my pregnancy." But she didn't worry too much. "My top priority was to have a healthy baby," she says. "I knew that my body would take care of the rest."

WINNING ACTION

Establish your personal calorie budget. When you're pregnant, your body needs extra calories to support your growing baby. But eating too much just might leave you with too many postpregnancy pounds. If you set up a calorie budget, like Karisa did, it can help guide your food choices throughout the day. Your doctor can help you determine the right number of calories that will nourish your baby and keep your weight gain within a healthy range.

SHE ATE FOR THREE—
AND LOST THE WEIGHT

Expecting twins means doubling up on lots of things: two cribs, two high chairs, two car seats. It also means being twice as careful about your eating habits, so you don't gain twice as much weight as you should.

That was Stephanie Harrison's objective almost from the moment that she found out she was carrying not one baby but two. "When the ultrasound showed twins, I got excited, but my husband, Mick, practically went into shock," recalls the 25-year-old Leanyer, Australia, native. "About 24 hours later, he was excited, and I was in shock."

Once the news sank in, Stephanie realized that she could get huge if she wasn't careful. Her 5-foot-8, 132-pound body would need more calories to support her growing babies, but not a lot more. "I certainly didn't want to starve my babies," she says. "But I didn't want to blow up either."

Hoping to avoid months or even years of trying to shed her postpregnancy pounds, Stephanie began scrutinizing her eating habits. They were already fairly healthful, but Stephanie saw room for improvement. "I ate fish instead of red meat, since fish has less saturated fat and is a little easier to digest," she says. "I cut back on margarine, too."

Changes like these enabled Stephanie to take in the extra calories that she needed while keeping a lid on her prenatal weight gain. By the time she delivered twins Ashlee and Ethan in April 2000, she had put on a total of 50 pounds. That's a little more than the recommended amount, but it's still considered healthy.

And the extra weight certainly didn't stick around for long. Within 6 weeks of giving birth, Stephanie had lost 40 pounds of baby fat. Breastfeeding burned up a lot of calories and pounds. But eating healthfully and walking regularly, with Ashlee and Ethan in their stroller, undoubtedly helped as well. "Just caring for two babies means I'm twice as active as if I'd had one," she says.

Stephanie would like to lose 15 more pounds, which would take her below her prepregnancy weight of 132. She concedes that she has to work harder to make good food choices: "Since having the twins, I find myself grabbing whatever I can, and unfortunately, it isn't always nutritious." For this reason, she's even more thankful that she took such good care of herself during her pregnancy. "Eating well while I was pregnant definitely gave me a head start on slimming down afterward," she says. "It has put my goal weight within reach."

W I N N I N G   A C T I O N

Expecting twins? Meet your calorie quota with the right foods. *If you're carrying twins, your body needs about 300 more calories a day than it would to adequately nourish just one baby. That may seem like a lot, but the calories can add up quickly, depending on your food choices. In general, many of the foods with the lowest calorie contents—like fruits and vegetables—also have the highest nutritional value. So the more of them you eat, the more vitamins and minerals you'll be supplying for your babies, but without excessively expanding your waistline.*

FOR THIS MOM-TO-BE, FINDING MOTIVATION WAS NO STRETCH

Between the persistent cravings and the lack of energy for exercise, staying fit during pregnancy can test the determination of any woman. That was the case for Laura Callahan. But when she needed to fire up her inspiration, she looked to an unusual place: her thighs.

At 5 feet 5 and 130 pounds, Laura was in great shape when she became pregnant with her first child in July 1997. But years before, as a college freshman, she had struggled with her weight. "You've heard of the freshman 15? For me, it was more like 35," says the 31-year-old Northbrook, Illinois, resident. "And most of those pounds seemed to go straight to my thighs."

Indeed, the weight accumulated so fast that at the tender age of 18, Laura found herself with stretch marks on her inner and outer thighs. Taking aerobics classes and walking helped her to lose the extra pounds. Once she got married, she stayed in shape by inline skating alongside her husband while he ran.

For 5 years, Laura's bathroom scale didn't budge above 130 pounds. Unfortunately, her stretch marks didn't budge either. So when she became pregnant, she had incentive to keep her weight gain within a healthy range. "No matter what, I was not about to get stretch marks on my stomach," she recalls.

With her doctor's okay, Laura began stationary biking and walking twice a week, and swimming once a week. She also started drinking lots of water, not only to stay hydrated but also to control her cravings.

By the time her daughter Emily arrived in May 1998, Laura had put on an extra 40 pounds—a healthy gain, according to her doctor. "And I had only one tiny stretch mark, underneath my stomach," she says. "I didn't even notice it right away."

Laura resumed her fitness program soon after Emily was born, walking 4 or 5 days a week with her daughter in tow. She also continued drinking lots of water, which helped control her appetite. Within 4 months, she lost an impressive 45 pounds—even more than she had gained during her pregnancy. "And that stretch mark on my stomach disappeared!" she says proudly.

Today, Laura is still holding steady at a fit and trim 125 pounds.

"I'm really proud of what I accomplished," she says. "If I get pregnant again, I'm confident that I could keep my weight gain under control."

WINNING ACTION

Stay in shape to steer clear of stretch marks. Stretch marks and pregnancy seem to go hand in hand. In fact, experts say that stretch marks—which occur when a protein called collagen separates from the skin's elastic fibers—can be prevented. The key is to manage your weight gain through a combination of good nutrition and regular physical activity. All the more reason to eat right and exercise throughout your pregnancy.

What if—despite your best efforts—you end up with stretch marks anyway? As Laura discovered, just slimming down may make the marks less noticeable, if not disappear completely.

THE POUNDS STAYED AWAY WHEN SHE PUT BABY FIRST

Motherhood didn't come easy for Mary Rose Sullivan. So when the Sacramento native finally became pregnant in June 1993, she did everything that she could to ensure a smooth pregnancy and a healthy start in life for her baby. Her efforts paid off, with an unexpected dividend: She gained just 25 pounds of baby fat—and lost every ounce.

Mary and her husband, Tim, very much wanted to have a child.

But because Mary had undergone surgery that required the removal of her fallopian tubes, she knew that in vitro fertilization offered her only hope for pregnancy. The procedure worked, but it kept her off her feet for several days. In fact, she wasn't allowed to resume her regular activity level until after her 13th week, a normal waiting period for women who have undergone in vitro fertilization.

Once she got the all clear from her doctor, Mary went back to her usual routine. She even did some low-impact exercise, just as she had before she became pregnant. It was a turning point for the ecstatic mom-to-be. "My priorities shifted," she explains. "I had been heavy in high school, so at first my main concern was to not regain the pounds I had worked so hard to lose. But when I found out that I was really going to be a mom, I became as determined to stay healthy for my baby as I had once been to control my weight."

For Mary, staying healthy meant eating nutritiously and engaging in regular physical activity to avoid adding too many pounds to her 5-foot-9½, 135-pound body. She reduced her fat consumption and reserved sweets as special treats. She phased out her favorite comfort foods—mashed potatoes, desserts, and fast food—in favor of healthier choices that would benefit her baby. She began walking on a daily basis, in addition to working out two or three times a week with some low-impact aerobics videos developed especially for moms-to-be.

Because of early dilation, Mary had to stop exercising for the last month of her pregnancy. No matter. Her healthy habits had already laid the groundwork for a successful delivery, not to mention rapid postpartum weight loss. Her 25 pounds of baby fat were gone within a few months of daughter Emma's arrival in March 1994.

For Mary, who's now 37, even more important than slimming down to her prepregnancy weight was giving birth to a beautiful little girl. Mary committed herself to a sound prenatal lifestyle, and both mother and daughter are healthier for it. "I've managed to keep my weight at 135 pounds, mostly through exercise," she says. "I've even gotten my black belt in karate!"

WINNING ACTION

Think about taking care of your body for your baby. *Concern about prenatal weight gain may not always be enough to dissuade you from caving in to a craving or forgoing your fitness routine. In those moments when you feel your motivation waning, ask yourself: "How will my actions affect my pregnancy?" Your answer may persuade you to make the healthy choice. Everything that you do to protect and support your baby will benefit you as well.*

SHE PARED POUNDS BY BECOMING PORTION-SAVVY

To lose weight, most people believe that they must cut calories or count grams of fat. Both strategies can help. But controlling portion sizes is equally important. Just ask first-time mom Jill Perrin. By learning to measure the amount of food on her plate, she did more than shed her 18 pounds of baby fat. She also overcame gestational diabetes, a potentially serious prenatal disease.

In the summer of 1998, when Jill and her husband found out that they were going to be parents, their excitement was matched by their anxiety. "Even though we had been married for 5 years, we hadn't planned on becoming pregnant," explains Jill, a 29-year-old market research analyst from Lowell, Massachusetts. "We had to get used to the fact that we were having a baby, ready or not."

As if the prospect of being parents wasn't daunting enough, the pregnancy would soon present its own hurdle. Through the first several months, Jill ate well, and she walked three or four times a week. Then the fatigue kicked in. Worse, Jill began experiencing insatiable cravings for sweets. "My blood sugar has always been unbalanced, so I try to avoid sugary foods like candy and baked goods," she says. "By my sixth month, I wanted them all the time."

Jill mentioned her symptoms to her obstetrician, who ran a blood test for gestational diabetes. It came back positive. "Honestly, I wasn't all that surprised," she says. "My sister had gestational diabetes, and diabetes runs in my family."

In moms-to-be with gestational diabetes, the pancreas can't make enough of the hormone insulin, which enables the body to convert blood sugar into energy. Left unchecked, the excess blood sugar can cross the placenta and affect the health of the baby.

To treat the disease, Jill's obstetrician sent her to a nutritionist, who put her on a 2,200-calorie-a-day diet and taught her to monitor her portion sizes. "I realized that I was eating way too much of everything, especially pasta," she says. One serving of pasta is just ½ cup, according to the USDA Food Guide Pyramid. "I was eating at least three!" she confesses.

The nutritionist also advised Jill to engage in regular physical activity, which helps the body use up excess blood sugar without needing extra insulin. Unfortunately, the bitter New England winter prevented Jill from exercising as much as she should have. But she made sure to stick with her diet, keeping a close eye on her portion sizes. "I didn't want to harm my baby just because I couldn't pass up a doughnut!" she says.

Jill's vigilance paid off: By the time she delivered her daughter, Maeve, in May 1999, she had added just 18 pounds to her 5-foot-6, 210-pound frame. She continued to eat healthfully while breastfeeding her baby. At her 6-week postpartum checkup, she got the news that her gestational diabetes had subsided. As a bonus, she was 10 pounds *below* her prepregnancy weight.

While Jill would like to be thinner, that's not her top priority. Her focus is on being a positive role model for Maeve. "Having a daughter has made me very aware that my self-image will shape how she thinks of herself," she says. "I want to raise a daughter who is confident and healthy, who feels good about her body."

W I N N I N G   A C T I O N

Remember that portion size matters. *Even healthy foods can pack on pounds if you eat too much of them. So pay attention to the serving sizes on food labels—and remember that if you consume more than the recommended serving, you're taking in extra calories and grams of fat. For foods that don't have labels, or for situations where you can't measure (in restaurants, for example), use these comparisons to eyeball your portions.*

- *Palm of one hand = 3 ounces of meat*
- *Thumb = 1 ounce of cheese*
- *Computer mouse = ½ cup of potatoes or pasta*
- *Tennis ball = 1 medium apple or orange*

Note: If you've been told that you have gestational diabetes, don't change your diet or other aspects of your treatment plan without consulting your physician. He knows your situation best and can offer advice tailored to your unique nutritional and medical needs.

CUTTING CALORIES LEADS TO UNEXPECTED POSTPREGNANCY PERK

Within a period of 4 months, Stacey Stevens lost her job and found out that she was pregnant. She credits both events with changing her lifestyle for the better. Her scale backs her up: Six months after her son, Brendan, was born, she had taken off 25 pounds of post-pregnancy baby fat *plus* 20 pounds of prepregnancy weight.

Before she became a mom-to-be, Stacey worked full-time as a marketing director for an Internet company. "The entire industry has a 'work hard, party hard' atmosphere," explains the 35-year-old Sonoma, California, resident. "My colleagues and I would eat out a lot—big meals, with appetizers, entrées, and desserts. I drank quite a bit, too—four to six beers over the course of an evening."

Stacey was enjoying herself so much that she scarcely noticed the pounds creeping on. "I'm 5 feet 11, so I can carry a lot of weight," she says. "Even at my heaviest, 190 pounds, I didn't look fat."

Then in April 1998, Stacey's company folded. "My coworkers and I still hung out together, but as people got jobs, we saw less and less of each other," she says. "I didn't go back to work, because my husband and I had decided to try to get pregnant. That really cut back on my socializing—and my eating and drinking."

Four months later, in August 1998, Stacey and her husband got the news they had been waiting for: They were going to be parents. Stacey, who had been treating herself to an occasional glass of wine, swore off alcohol for good, knowing that it could do devastating harm to her growing baby. She also kept junk food out of her house. "I have a big problem with portion control," she admits. "If I start eating something, I'll keep at it until it's gone. So I decided to avoid the temptation by not having those foods around."

Through her pregnancy, Stacey gained a healthy 25 pounds. She began losing shortly after giving birth to Brendan in April 1999. "I expected to get rid of the baby fat because I was nursing," she says. "But I hit my prepregnancy weight and just kept going." Six months later, she had taken off a total of 45 pounds.

While some of her weight loss could be attributed to breastfeeding, Stacey believed that something else had enabled her to shed all those extra pounds. Then it hit her: Between giving up alcohol and eating fewer extravagant meals, she was saving herself hundreds—if not thousands—of calories a week.

With a second baby on the way, Stacey is even more motivated to maintain her healthy lifestyle. And not just to control her prenatal weight gain. "My son is old enough to see me as an example," she says. "I need to do a better job for his sake."

WINNING ACTION

Check your diet for empty calories. When you're pregnant, your body needs extra calories to sustain and nourish your growing baby. But if you're getting those calories from the wrong sources, you could be setting yourself up for excessive weight gain—and putting your baby at risk.

In Stacey's case, giving up alcohol is one of the best things she could have done for herself and her son. Alcohol can cause serious birth defects in developing fetuses. It also contains an abundance of empty calories that really pack on the pounds. Every time Stacey drank four to six beers, she was taking in an extra 600 to 900 calories. At that rate, she could have been putting on a pound a week (3,500 calories equals 1 pound).

Of course, the most important reason not to consume alcohol during pregnancy is to protect your baby. Switch to other refreshing, low-calorie drinks such as flavored seltzer water and unsweetened iced tea. Be sure to drink plenty of water and fat-free milk as well.

20 POUNDS GONE—2 WEEKS AFTER DELIVERING TWINS

You might say that Julie Brooks Hiller was a late bloomer. At age 35, she took up running. One year later, she became pregnant—with twins. But that didn't slow her down. In fact, it gave her even more incentive to stay in shape.

Julie first became interested in running as a means of firming up her 5-foot-4, 105-pound physique. "Even though I had never experienced a weight problem, I wanted to hang on to my 'bikini body,'" explains the East Coventry, Pennsylvania, native. "Running not only kept me slim and firm, it gave me greater strength and stamina. I liked that."

These benefits would work to Julie's advantage when she became pregnant in February 1996. As her doctor explained, the risks associated with pregnancy become even greater as a woman gets older. That went double for Julie, since she was carrying twins.

Julie took her doctor's cautions seriously, but she believed that being fit would help to see her through a healthy pregnancy and a problem-free delivery. "I didn't even worry about my weight," she says. "I convinced myself that if I could just stay active, my body would take care of the rest."

At first, Julie stuck with running, putting in 3 miles a day—consistent with her prepregnancy workout. Then when she was 2 months along, her doctor advised her to find an activity that was less jarring. She began swimming in her backyard pool for an hour a day and walking as often as she could.

"My doctor also gave me a handout with exercises to strengthen my abdominal and back muscles, which I practiced for 7 months," Julie says. "They helped prepare my body for the weight of the babies and for the demands of delivery."

Julie's commitment to prenatal exercise paid off. She looked fit and felt great throughout her pregnancy, even avoiding the persistent fatigue that affects so many moms-to-be. "Remember, I had been running 3 miles a day," she says. "My body was accustomed to being put through its paces."

By the time she gave birth to Sean and Wesley in October 1996, Julie had gained only 32 pounds, slightly less than is typical for a new mom of twins. And she began losing the extra weight almost immediately, taking off approximately 20 pounds in just 2 weeks and another 5 soon after. To what does she owe the quick return of her prepregnancy physique? Regular exercise, plain and simple.

"I believe that I had no weight problem during or after my pregnancy because I was fit *before* I got pregnant and I remained active until my sons were born," says Julie, who at age 40 is holding steady at 112 pounds. "Now my sons help me stay in shape. There's no better workout than keeping up with two 4½-year-old boys!"

WINNING ACTION

Stay active from the start of your pregnancy. *Maintaining a moderate level of physical activity throughout your pregnancy can help you manage your weight gain* *and make those postpartum pounds melt away quickly. Research has shown that staying active can also shorten labor; improve stamina before, during, and after delivery; reduce the need for obstetric interventions; and speed recovery following childbirth.*

If you've been exercising regularly, your doctor can help you make appropriate adjustments in your fitness routine as your pregnancy progresses. If you've been relatively inactive, your doctor can help you establish an appropriate prenatal workout. Be sure to follow your doctor's advice: Some exercises, such as situps, are not recommended for moms-to-be.

PSSST! *THIS MOM'S WEIGHT-LOSS SECRET IS OUT*

Jennifer Love has a unique way of getting back into shape after pregnancy: She trains for triathlons. It's demanding, but so far, it has helped her to control her prenatal weight gain and shed a total of 70 postpregnancy pounds.

Jennifer's biggest concern has always been that she'll get cold feet and back out of an event. Since she relies on her training to regain her prepregnancy physique, withdrawing could have a serious effect on her waistline, not to mention her bathroom scale. So the 33-year-old Wilmington, Delaware, resident has come up with the perfect strategy to stop her from bailing out. "I tell my friends that I'm going to be competing," she says. "That way, I have to do it!"

Not that Jennifer's friends pressure her to follow through. Just

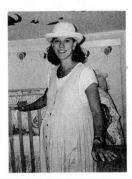

5 months pregnant

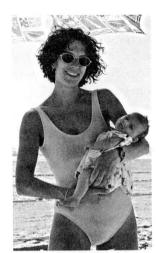

2 months after delivery

the fact that they know what she's up to gives her incentive to keep training. "I'd be too embarrassed to chicken out," she admits.

Once she has announced her intentions, Jennifer heads for the gym, where she works out for an hour, 5 days a week. She does make some adjustments in her workouts, switching to less "bouncy" activities while she's pregnant. "I swim and use the cross-trainer more often, and I walk instead of running on the treadmill," she says. "I continue to exercise until the day that I deliver."

This regimen enables Jennifer to stay fit through pregnancy, so she doesn't need to lose much weight afterward. It also gives her the best odds of being ready by race day.

It certainly seems to be working. During each of her first two pregnancies, Jennifer, who's 5 feet 7, gained only 35 pounds. She lost the weight within months of delivering Michaelie, who's now 3, and Sydney, who's 2. Once back to her prepregnancy weight of 135, she was ready for competition.

After the birth of her third daughter, Jamie, who's 8 months, Jennifer set her sights on her next triathlon. In all the years that she has been competing, she has yet to miss an event. Still, she says, "I don't consider myself a hard-core athlete at all. I do it for fun and for motivation."

WINNING ACTION

Inform family and friends of your intentions. *Even if you're not about to enter a triathlon, you can benefit from telling those closest to you about your plans to manage your prenatal weight gain. Once they know, they'll be able to lend their support to your efforts. Maybe your mom will rethink baking you a batch of your favorite chocolate chip cookies. Perhaps your husband will ask you to go for a postdinner stroll. These small gestures can make a big difference in whether or not you achieve your goal. They'll also motivate you to hold up your end of the bargain.*

HER NEW STRATEGY FOR SNACKING HELPED MELT AWAY BABY FAT

As much as Tia Scammahorn looked forward to motherhood, she dreaded the prospect of prenatal weight gain. At 5 feet 2 and 190 pounds, the St. Paul, Minnesota, mom-to-be didn't want to get heavier, for fear that the baby fat would become permanent. In fact, she had just started exercising regularly shortly before finding out that she was pregnant. Yet 2 months after delivery, she was back to her prepregnancy weight and eager to lose even more.

At the start of her pregnancy, Tia was told that because she already had some extra pounds to support her baby, she wouldn't need to put on as much as other moms-to-be. "My doctor said that if I went up to 200 pounds, I'd be fine," she recalls.

Tia was relieved by that news. After all, she reasoned, 10 pounds would be easier to lose than 25 to 35, the typical prenatal weight gain. But she also realized that she'd have to change her eating habits in order to stay within her doctor's recommendation.

"I never considered myself an overeater," Tia explains. "But I had a tendency to make poor food choices, especially when I was in a rush. I'd grab a quick snack at a fast-food restaurant or a convenience store."

Stopping at these places may have saved Tia time, but it didn't spare her fat or calories. If only eating healthfully were more convenient, she thought. That gave her an idea: She'd stock her own kitchen with nutritious foods that she could carry along and eat when she felt hungry. "I chose easy items like juices, soups, and some of the more convenient-to-carry nutrition bars," Tia notes. "I also tried to have regular meals at home, so I'd be less tempted to stop somewhere after work or while out running errands."

By making these minor adjustments in her eating habits, Tia managed to keep her prenatal weight gain to 15 pounds—more than her doctor recommended, but still within a healthy range. She gave birth to daughter Sophia in December 1999, then lost all of her baby fat within 2 months.

Tia believes that she was able to slim down so quickly in part because she was breastfeeding, in part because she had trimmed her consumption of high-fat, high-calorie convenience foods. At age 24, she's more optimistic than ever that she can finally shed her extra pounds. She'd like to slim down to 150. "I think that I have a better handle on what I need to be doing," she says. "And, of course, I have Sophia. She's my motivation for wanting to be fit and healthy."

WINNING ACTION

Make healthful food choices convenient. *When you're on the run, you're more inclined to succumb to impulse food purchases, like a candy bar at the drugstore or nachos with cheese at the mall. You end up spending a sizable portion of your day's fat and calorie allotment on foods with virtually no nutritional value for you or your baby. If you're prone to spur-of-the-moment munchies, you can prepare for them by stocking up on healthy choices, such as snack-size boxes of raisins and cereals, cans of low-sodium vegetable juice cocktail, and small bags of whole-wheat pretzels. Keep them in your purse, your glove compartment, your desk drawer—wherever they'll be handy when hunger strikes.*

DOCTOR'S ORDERS MADE HER TOE THE LINE ON EATING

When Leah Flickinger received word that she was a mom-to-be, the 35-year-old Lehigh Valley, Pennsylvania, resident vowed that she would have a healthy pregnancy. Then her hormones took over.

"Food was the only thing that seemed to combat my morning

sickness," she recalls. "Every time I felt a wave of nausea, I would eat." Exercising proved to be a challenge, too. She felt so exhausted that whenever she had time to work out, she wanted to nap instead.

The combination of eating more and exercising less quickly took its toll: Leah added 15 pounds to her 5-foot-8, 128-pound frame in just the first 3 months of her pregnancy. "I was ready for maternity pants by the end of the first trimester!" she laughs.

During her second trimester, Leah mustered enough energy to walk for a half-hour several times a week. But she couldn't free herself from her fixation on food. "I constantly made excuses to eat more," she says. "I needed milkshakes for calcium, a bagel with my breakfast cereal to get me through my half-hour commute, and snacks all day long to maintain my energy." By her seventh month, she weighed 158 pounds.

That's when Leah got a big dose of reality. "My ob-gyn actually scolded me for gaining too much weight, saying that it could cause complications," she recalls. Leah realized that if she kept up her excessive eating, her baby might grow too large for her narrow frame, increasing her chances of needing a cesarean section. "The last thing I wanted was to be recovering from major surgery while figuring out how to care for a newborn," Leah says.

So she took action. Rather than eating whatever and whenever she wanted, she put more thought into making healthy food choices. She gave up her 344-calorie breakfast bagel with cream cheese, replacing it with a 78-calorie hard-boiled egg—and saving 266 calories. Likewise, she traded in her 8-ounce chocolate milkshake for 8 ounces of low-fat milk, saving another 167 calories. Her portion sizes became smaller, too. "As the baby got bigger, I had less room in my stomach for large meals," she explains.

The day she gave birth to her daughter, Willa, in February 1999, Leah weighed in at 166 pounds. By reining in her eating habits (and maintaining her walking routine), she gained only 8 more pounds during her last trimester, and a manageable 38 pounds for the entire pregnancy. Best of all, her baby fat disappeared within 6 months. "Breastfeeding helped, because it burns a lot of calories," she says. "But being more conscientious about my food choices was just as important."

WINNING ACTION

Pay attention to what you're putting in your mouth. *Some women subscribe to the philosophy that while they're pregnant, they can eat whatever they crave, because that's what their bodies need. Yet, they should be even more vigilant about their food choices, because everything that goes in their mouths can affect their growing babies—for better or for worse. So think twice about what you're eating. Even consider keeping a food journal to monitor your dietary habits. In the long run, you and your baby will be healthier for your efforts.*

MIGHTY MOMS SAVED HER PREPREGNANCY FIGURE

"I love Mighty Moms!" Connie Osborn exclaims. No, the 28-year-old Tallahassee, Florida, resident isn't talking about some new breed of superhero. Mighty Moms is the pregnancy preparedness class that helped Connie hold her prenatal weight gain to 20 pounds—and lose those pounds almost immediately after delivery.

Connie found out about Mighty Moms when she was 3½

months into her second pregnancy. At the time, she was worried that her prenatal weight gain might get out of control. "When I got pregnant with my first son, Chandler, who's now 6, I was waitressing—a very physical job," she explains. "I put on 20 pounds with him, but they came off quickly.

"During my second pregnancy, I was working as a bookkeeper/office manager. I basically sat on my butt all day. I was afraid that my inactive lifestyle might really pack on the pounds, especially since I was 6 years older than when I had Chandler."

These concerns were hovering in the back of Connie's mind the day she walked into a consignment shop and found a business card for Mighty Moms, a fitness program designed especially for moms-to-be. "I was so excited," she recalls. "As soon as I got my doctor's approval, I signed up."

The classes met for 2 hours once a week, during which Connie and her fellow Mighty Moms were put through the paces by Michelle Holzman, a labor and delivery nurse and certified fitness trainer. Holzman had developed the prenatal fitness program, which featured lunges, modified pushups, modified abdominal exercises (tensing and holding the ab muscles), and strength training, in addition to relaxation techniques.

Connie found the classes to be a real challenge. "It definitely wasn't about pampering," she says. "We worked hard." But she noticed the results, primarily in the form of increased energy and improved muscle tone. "Even when I was 9 months pregnant, I felt good, and I could walk around just fine," she says.

In fact, Connie took her last Mighty Moms class just 3 days before delivering her second son, Devin, in March 2000. "My labor was better than textbook," she says. "I had such control over what I was doing. I pushed three times, and the baby was out!" She didn't even need an episiotomy, unlike her first delivery.

The day she left the hospital with her son, Connie—who's 5 feet 8—weighed in at 135 pounds. Within the week, she was back to her prepregnancy weight of 133.

Connie's positive experience with Mighty Moms has inspired her to continue working out on a regular basis. Even her husband, who she says never picked up a weight in his life, loves to join her at the gym. "He's looking better than ever," she adds. "And I'm in better shape than before I had my babies!"

WINNING ACTION

Sign up for a prenatal fitness program. *Many hospitals, health clubs, and YM/YWCAs offer exercise classes designed especially for moms-to-be. These classes not only help you control your pregnancy weight gain but also give you strength and energy for labor and delivery. Many women value the mental and emotional lift that comes from spending time with other moms-to-be.*

Ask your doctor about prenatal fitness programs that may be offered in your area. Of course, you should get your doctor's approval before launching an exercise routine during pregnancy.

THIS MOM USED THE BUDDY SYSTEM TO SLIM DOWN

If Becky Christy had one thing to do over, she'd be more careful about her eating habits during her pregnancy with daughter Caitlin, who's now 4. Between overeating and giving up exercise, she put on 45 pounds—weight that took her more than 2 years to lose.

"I was so excited about being a mom that I really wanted to look pregnant," explains the 33-year-old Madison, Wisconsin, resident. "I wasn't eating 'bad' foods. But I ate way too much."

So when she found out that she was expecting again, Becky vowed to take better care of herself. And she did, with a little help from a friend.

Becky met Jennifer Rae in late 1998. Their husbands worked together, and the two women became quite close. Coincidentally, they became pregnant at about the same time—Becky first, Jennifer a few months later.

Together, the two women planned how they would manage their prenatal weight gain so that their pregnancies would be healthy and trouble-free. They continued working out at their respective gyms for as long as they could. Becky's routine consisted of 30 minutes of cardiovascular exercise four to five times a week, plus strength training for 30 minutes, three times a week. "My husband, Dan, went to the gym with me and spotted for me while I was lifting weights," she says. "I couldn't have continued my workouts without him."

With support from both her husband and her friend, Becky held her prenatal weight gain to 30 pounds—appropriate for her 5-foot-4½, 138-pound body. She easily lost 24 of those pounds within 2 months of delivery, primarily because she had stayed active through most of her pregnancy.

Once Jennifer had her baby, the bond between the two women grew even stronger. Both were keeping journals, and they met once a week to make sure that their weight-loss efforts stayed on track. "Jennifer helped me a lot with maintaining a healthy lifestyle," Becky says.

With daughter Cassidy now a year old, Becky is still working on losing the last of her postpregnancy pounds. "I've even created my own diet-and-exercise plan to help me slim down," Becky says. She's still keeping her journal, and she and Jennifer still get together once a week to compare notes. And, of course, they brag about their babies, too!

WINNING ACTION

Seek support from other moms-to-be. *No one understands the intricacies of pregnancy better than a woman who's expecting. If you know of someone with a baby on the way—a family member, friend, or coworker, for example—talk with her about becoming "pregnancy buddies." You can coach and support each other through challenges big and small, including managing your prenatal weight gain.*

SOY SAVED HER FROM PERMANENT BABY FAT

When 35-year-old New York City resident Julie Boehning became a vegan, she did it out of social consciousness, not health consciousness. But her decision to give up all animal products would have a profound, positive impact on her physical well-being. Ultimately, it would play a significant role in helping her get into shape after the birth of her son, Julian.

Julie adopted veganism in the early 1990s, after years of being an ovo-lactovegetarian (meaning that she ate eggs and dairy, but no other animal products). Her outrage over the actions of an agricultural company had persuaded her to give up dairy products. "I wanted to take a stand," she says. "It was my little protest against a big business."

Her transition to veganism was not without challenges. Julie knew that she needed to find alternative sources of the essential proteins provided by meats and dairy products. She had to be sure to get all of her vitamins and minerals, too, since she couldn't digest large multivitamins. Her search eventually led her to soy and soy products.

"I discovered that soy foods taste really good," she says. "Some of my favorites are tofu, tempeh, and soy cheese, yogurt, and milk. But so many great-tasting soy products are available these days."

Before long, Julie noticed that her new style of eating was producing some unexpected health benefits. Most notably, the rheumatoid arthritis pain that had plagued her since she was a teenager began to subside. "I used to walk with a limp, which really irritated me," she says. "Miraculously, it went away. But I didn't connect my recovery to my new eating habits—at least not at first." Then she came across an article suggesting that a meatless diet could be an effective treatment for rheumatoid arthritis.

When Julie became pregnant in December 1998, she saw no reason to forsake veganism. Her doctor reassured her that a well-balanced vegan diet would support her and her growing baby's nutritional needs. And as long as she made the effort to eat lots of soy foods, she would get all the protein she needed to support her pregnancy. Indeed, building her meals around soy and other plant-based foods likely helped Julie limit her prenatal weight gain to 35 pounds—healthy for her 5-foot-4, 103-pound body.

The benefits of veganism became even more evident to Julie after she gave birth to Julian in September 1999. Once a runner and a regular at the local gym, she found herself forgoing her daily workouts. "I had a cesarean section, and my physical activity was really limited for about 6 weeks afterward," she recalls. "By then I was so busy with the baby that I had no time to run or go to the gym to exercise."

Even without a fitness routine, Julie began slimming down rather quickly. "What I ate really helped a lot," she says. What did she eat? A balanced diet consisting primarily of fruits, vegetables, whole grain breads, beans, and, of course, soy foods.

Within 10 months of delivering her son, Julie lost 27 of her post-pregnancy pounds. Her goal is to return to 103, her prepregnancy weight. "I have 8 pounds to go, and I'm confident that my vegan diet will get me there," she says. "It has done so much for me already!"

WINNING ACTION

Make soy a dietary staple. *Soy is an excellent choice for both moms-to-be and breastfeeding moms because it's a complete protein—in other words, it contains all nine essential amino acids, just like meat and dairy products. But it's much lower in fat than animal-derived foods. Most supermarkets now carry an array of soy foods, from soy milk and soy cheese to soy burgers and soy sausage. Sample different products to find some that you like, then use them for occasional meat-free, dairy-free meals.*

MODERATION, NOT DEPRIVATION, REINED IN HER PRENATAL GAIN

Dana Bacher's favorite nightcap is ice cream. She helps herself to a small cup every evening, just as she did during her pregnancy. And she weighs less now than before she became a mom.

Lest you think that the 29-year-old Macungie, Pennsylvania, resident is blessed with a super-speedy metabolism, you should

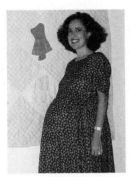

5 days before delivery

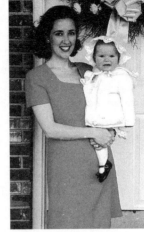

7 months after delivery

know that she struggled with her weight all through her teenage years. Dana was a dancer—and quite weight-conscious. "I was always 10 to 15 pounds heavier than I should have been," she says. "I tried all kinds of extreme diets—the ones I would see in women's magazines, like the grapefruit diet and the rice diet. I wanted so badly to slim down, but nothing seemed to work."

Within a year of graduating from college, Dana became so frustrated and disillusioned by her inability to lose weight that she just quit dieting and began eating normal foods, with the exception of meat, which she had given up during her junior year. To her surprise, the pounds gradually melted from her petite 5-foot frame. She eventually dropped down to 98 pounds.

Dana realized that she didn't need to deprive herself of food in order to be trim and healthy. She could eat what she wanted, like cheese and pasta, as long as she didn't go overboard with second helpings. "I discovered moderation, and that really made a difference for me," she says.

This lesson worked to Dana's advantage when she became pregnant for the first time. Rather than panicking about prenatal weight gain, she redoubled her efforts to eat healthfully, but without denying herself anything. "I was hungry for 'cool' foods, like ice cream and salads, and foods that I don't normally eat, like sandwiches from Subway," she says. "I indulged these cravings, but I was very careful to limit serving sizes."

Dana did increase the size of her regular meals ever so slightly, to support her growing baby. To avoid light-headedness, she ate breakfast every morning—something she had never done routinely in her adult life. She also began walking regularly, once a day at first, and twice a day later on.

Dana's strategy worked wonderfully. She gained a healthy 25 pounds before giving birth to daughter Katie in August 1998. She lost all of the baby fat within a year. She believes that she achieved weight-loss success at least in part because she eats what she wants, in moderation.

"I don't exclude anything from my diet, because that leads to cravings, and cravings will only make me overeat in the long run," Dana says. "I'll have what I'm hungry for, but I'll keep the portion small. And I'll eat it slowly, so I can really enjoy it!"

WINNING ACTION

Indulge your prenatal cravings without guilt. *Some experts theorize that moms-to-be develop cravings for certain foods as their bodies try to shore up nutritional support for their growing babies. Of course, you're more likely to get a hankering for potato chips than carrots, or chocolate than cherries. In that case, you may be better off eating what you want instead of searching for a healthy substitute. Just remember to control the portion* *size. For example, grab a handful of chips or a single snack-size candy bar, then put the rest of the bag away. And eat slowly, to truly savor each bite.*

THIS MOM'S EXERCISE ROUTINE MAKES A SPLASH

After being diagnosed with multiple sclerosis in 1994, Catharine Keyes took up swimming as a means of staying fit both physically and mentally. She didn't know it at the time, but her activity of choice would also help her to manage her prenatal weight gain and take off 30 postpregnancy pounds.

When Catharine began treatment for multiple sclerosis (MS), she had a tough time coping with the disease. "I was taking prednisone, I had stopped exercising, and I probably wasn't eating all that well either," recalls the Madison, New Jersey, resident. All three factors conspired to add 60 pounds to her 5-foot-10, 160-pound frame over the course of a year.

The dramatic weight gain convinced Catharine that she had to make some changes in her lifestyle. With help from a registered dietitian, she cleaned up her eating habits. She also started swimming, following the advice of her neurologist and a physical therapist. Within a year, she lost the 60 extra pounds.

Swimming proved to be the perfect exercise for Catharine. "I used to walk a couple of miles at a time, but it was hard," she says. "My body temperature would rise, and because of MS's effects on my nerves, I'd develop leg cramps and fatigue." With swimming, Catharine didn't have to worry about any of that. "It cooled my body while providing a workout similar to walking, in terms of calorie burn and aerobic fitness," she explains.

Her passion for the pool would grow even more important when Catharine became pregnant in 1998. Remembering how swimming had helped her slim down before, she decided that it could also help her avoid putting on too much baby fat. She continued her exercise routine—one mile (40 minutes) in the pool three times a week—for the duration of her pregnancy. She gained just 32 pounds before giving birth to son Robert in May 1999.

Catharine wasted no time getting back in the pool. She resumed her swimming routine almost immediately after delivery. Six months later, she had dropped 30 of her postpregnancy pounds. She has kept them off ever since.

Now 34, Catharine continues to swim regularly. She still appreciates the sport's physical benefits, but she has come to value its mental and emotional benefits just as much. "I see it as a chance to treat myself," she says. "If I can't find 3 hours a week to do something for myself, in terms of my MS and my general health, then I need to reevaluate my priorities."

WINNING ACTION

Swim to achieve prenatal fitness. *For moms-to-be, most experts recommend physical activities that don't require bouncy, jerky movements. Swimming fills the bill perfectly. Its smooth, rhythmic strokes and kicks provide you with a good aerobic workout, while the water supports your body weight. It's a great form of exercise, especially for women who weren't all that active before their pregnancies. Many health clubs and YMCAs have aquatic facilities. Check around for hours and fees.*

BABY FAT GAVE HER FOOD FOR THOUGHT

As a fitness instructor, Connie Warasila feels a special obligation to take care of her body and set a good example for her students. As a mother of two, she understands the unique challenges of staying in shape during pregnancy. After all, she ballooned by more than 50 pounds while pregnant with her first child. With her second, she made a conscious effort not to let history repeat itself.

While many moms-to-be have a hard time getting enough exercise, that certainly wasn't the case for Connie. She continued teaching step aerobics, aqua aerobics, and other fitness classes through most of her two pregnancies. So why did she put on so many pounds during her first pregnancy? "I just ate too much," concedes the 36-year-old Annandale, Virginia, resident. "I had a special fondness for sweets, especially coconut cake."

Even working out regularly couldn't save Connie's 5-foot-8, 165-pound figure from her dietary indulgences. She gained 52 pounds while pregnant—as much as double what's usually considered healthy. But after delivering son Max in April 1997, she had special incentive to slim down quickly.

"I needed to lose the weight so that when I resumed my aerobics classes, my students could take me seriously and respect me as a fitness instructor," Connie explains. "Also, I couldn't show my students proper alignment and biomechanics if I was hiding my body under a big T-shirt."

Connie managed to slim down to her prepregnancy weight within 10 months of delivering Max. "I exercised consistently, drank lots of water, and limited my food portions until the pounds were gone," she says. Two years later, she became pregnant again. She couldn't help remembering what had happened to her figure the first time around. The second time would be different.

BRADFORD WG LIBRARY
100 HOLLAND COURT, BOX 130
BRADFORD ONT L3Z 2A7

"I became very careful about my eating habits," Connie explains. "I gave up sweets and empty carbohydrates, replacing them with fresh fruits and vegetables, whole grains, and lean protein. I drank a lot of water, too—128 ounces a day. That seemed to help."

Indeed, Connie kept her prenatal weight gain to 35 pounds, 17 pounds less than during her first pregnancy. The weight came off faster, too: She was back to her prepregnancy weight just 7 months after son Kevin's arrival in September 1999.

Connie is convinced that becoming a mom has changed her eating habits for the better. It has encouraged her to make other healthful adjustments in her lifestyle as well. "I drink less alcohol, and I get more sleep," she says. "I'm much more conscientious about my health. That's good for me, and it's good for my boys."

WINNING ACTION

Rewrite the "rules" from your previous pregnancies. If you've struggled to lose baby fat before, you may feel that you're destined for an even more difficult battle during your current pregnancy. But you can change your destiny simply by learning from the past. Think back to your first pregnancy and identify areas where you might make changes that are good for you and your baby. Maybe you didn't exercise as often as you should have, or perhaps you let your dietary habits slide because you were "eating for two." By recognizing and addressing these issues, you may be able to rein in your prenatal weight gain this time around.

FOR THIS MOM, SWEETS ARE TREATS, NOT CHEATS

For as long as she can remember, Cara Lemm has had a sweet tooth. She used to indulge it quite freely, eating candy, cake, and cookies whenever she got the urge. But when she and her husband decided to start a family, she knew that she would have to control her sugar habit. It would only contribute to her pregnancy weight gain—and that wouldn't be healthy for her or her babies.

Cara counted herself as one of the fortunate few whose propensity for sweets didn't threaten their waistlines. At 5 feet 7 and 125 pounds, she had always been naturally thin. "I had more of a problem maintaining my weight than gaining," explains the 31-year-old Austin, Texas, resident. "In fact, if I didn't eat enough, I'd start losing pretty quickly."

Some women only wish they had this problem! But Cara understood that pregnancy would dramatically change her body's nutritional needs. She also realized that after she had a baby, the pounds might not come off so easily.

So when she became pregnant for the first time, Cara established a new personal policy on sweets. "I could treat myself to dessert only if I ate a good, nutritious meal first," she says. "I started eating lots of veggies, usually with rice, noodles, or potatoes. I sometimes had meat, but I kept the portion small."

Cara's strategy worked, though not quite as she expected. "I found myself getting so full on the good stuff that I had less room for dessert," she says. "Even when I was hungry for something sweet, I didn't eat as much as I used to."

Cara, the self-described sugar addict, had successfully reined in her sweet tooth. She gained 19 pounds before giving birth to her first child, Travis, in June 1990. "And those pounds came off quickly, within 2 weeks, mostly because I was breastfeeding," she says.

Over the next 8 years, Cara had three more children—two boys, Tyler and Jason, and one girl, Grace. Through each pregnancy, she gained between 20 and 24 pounds. And she lost every one of those pounds—plus a few more. "After my third and fourth pregnancies, the weight hung on longer—up to 6 months," she says. "I suspect it's because I was older and I didn't have a lot of muscle tone."

Amazingly, Cara weighs less now than she did *before* she became a mom. She's convinced that her new-and-improved eating habits, which she has maintained ever since her first pregnancy, are responsible for her slim 118-pound physique. "Because I'm eating better, I'm setting a good example for my kids," she says. "Like me, they get dessert only if they eat a healthy meal first!"

WINNING ACTION

Save your sweets for postmeal treats. *Many women develop a sweet tooth during pregnancy, even if they never craved sugary foods before. Of course, denying yourself ice cream, candy bars, and baked goods only makes you want them more. So instead of just saying no, tell yourself that you can enjoy your treat after you've eaten something more nutritious. By then, your craving may be gone, or you may be content with a smaller portion. Either way, you'll feel satisfied rather than deprived.*

DINING OUT IS NO LONGER ON HER MENU

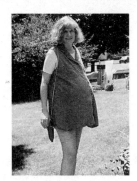

3 days before delivery

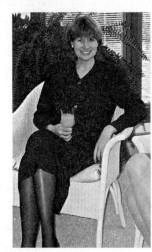

4 months after delivery

Pam and Brian Boyer loved to go out for dinner. And they did it routinely—as often as four nights a week. But when the couple found out that they'd be having twins, Pam began to re-think their restaurant ritual. She knew that the rich meals could spell trouble for her soon-to-be-growing waistline.

For the Boyers, eating out provided a welcome opportunity to kick back and unwind after a busy day. With restaurants plentiful near their Bethlehem, Pennsylvania, home, perhaps their biggest challenge was deciding where to go. Their tastes ran to seafood and Italian, though they would try just about anything.

With news of their pending parenthood, Pam realized that she had to be more particular about her food choices, especially from restaurant menus. She seized on the opportunity to improve her eating habits—for herself and her twins.

Gone were not only the rich seafood and Italian dishes from her dinners out but also the junk food and sweets. In their place, she ate lots of lean protein, fruits, and vegetables, and drank lots of milk. "I tried to do everything by the book because Brian and I had tried so hard to have these kids," she explains. "I did everything that I could to make sure that they'd be healthy."

Indeed, Adam and Sean couldn't have been any more perfect when they arrived in July 1999. As for Pam, she gained just 35 pounds through her pregnancy. And she lost all of it within 6 weeks of delivery, maintaining her 5-foot-6 body at 125 pounds ever since.

"I was surprised, because I really didn't have to struggle too much to take off or keep off the weight," she says. "I think the combination of not going out to dinner as often and being in constant motion really helped."

With the twins on the brink of toddlerhood, Pam—who's now 36—doesn't see herself and her husband resuming their restaurant ritual anytime soon. Not that she misses it. "Food was much more of a focal point in our lives before the babies," she says. "Now it's not so important anymore."

WINNING ACTION

Reserve restaurant meals for special occasions. *Eating out may soon rival baseball as America's national pastime. Sure, it's convenient. But when it becomes a habit, it can really take a toll on your waistline—just what you don't need when you're expecting. Even a dish that seems low in fat and calories can be unhealthy, because restaurant portions tend to be huge. Feel free to eat out, but avoid making it an everyday occurrence. And be sure to ask for a doggy bag, so you*

*can cut your entrée in half and take home the leftovers
for another meal.*

*THIS TIME, SHE WON'T BE
STRESSED BY BABY FAT*

Colleen Gibbs worked hard at staying fit and healthy, embracing
vegetarianism and exercising for 2 hours a day. Then she became
pregnant for the first time, just before the 1998 holiday season. Suddenly, the woman who had taken such pride in her body found herself eating not just for two but for an entire army.

Using her pending motherhood as an excuse to indulge,
Colleen dug into all of the traditional holiday gustatory delights
with gusto. Her refrigerator frequently housed a selection of
Christmas goodies such as mashed potatoes, cookies, and pudding.

And when the festive mealtimes rolled around, Colleen had a
hard time saying no to anything that passed in her direction.
"Having a pregnant woman at the table is a delicious novelty," notes
the 38-year-old Carlsbad, California, resident. "Everyone is saying,
'Eat this, have this, try this, you'll lose it later!' "

As her pregnancy progressed, Colleen began experiencing
major fatigue. She worked full-time as director of public relations
for an Internet firm. Some days she would get home, eat, and fall
asleep. She didn't have the time or the energy for exercise. "The only
thing that I was lifting was a fork," she laughs.

Between the overeating and the lack of exercise, it's a miracle
that Colleen gained only 30 pounds through her pregnancy. That's
right in the ballpark for someone who's 5 feet 3 and 120 pounds.

Still, the baby fat hung around longer than she expected after son Terence's arrival in January 1999. "The weight loss just wasn't happening for me," she says. "I remember thinking, 'It has to be because of all those unhealthy foods.'"

Eventually, Colleen did lose all 30 pounds, spurred on by sheer willpower and a strong ego. She stepped up her workouts, pared down her meals to healthy proportions, and drank lots of water. That experience taught Colleen a valuable lesson.

Now she's expecting her second child, and she's determined to make this pregnancy healthier than the first. She has already made one big change: Since becoming a parent, she's working part-time from her home instead of an office. This has freed up time for her to prepare healthful meals, to visit the gym regularly—and, of course, to chase after little Terence wherever they go.

Perhaps even more important than her new lifestyle is her new attitude. During her first pregnancy, Colleen would obsess about her weight gain, which made her eat even more. Now she accepts the pregnancy pounds as perfectly natural. She understands that they'll come off, provided she does her part by eating healthfully and exercising regularly.

"I'm not sweating the weight anywhere near as much as I did the last time," Colleen says. "I know that it's necessary to support my baby. And that's my ultimate goal: to have a healthy child."

WINNING ACTION

Accept prenatal weight gain, but don't make it an excuse. *When you're pregnant, your body gains as many pounds as it needs to support your growing baby. It will shed much of that weight soon after your baby is born. Nature will take care of everything, provided you do your part by practicing good prenatal nutrition and en-*

gaging in regular prenatal exercise—with your doctor's approval, of course. Pregnancy is a wondrous, miraculous experience. So don't stress about it. Celebrate it, marvel at it—and enjoy it!

THIS MOM CHANGED HER PERSPECTIVE ON PROTEIN

For Valerie Schultz, red meat and pending motherhood never mixed. The Tehachapi, California, mother of four simply lost her carnivorous cravings during her first three pregnancies. By her fourth, she had decided to go along with her body and give up red meat for good. In hindsight, she thinks that may have helped her rein in her prenatal weight gain.

Valerie used to enjoy a good steak dinner just as much as anyone. But when she became pregnant with daughter Morgan, who's now 18, she suddenly lost her appetite for red meat. "For whatever reason, it just didn't agree with me," she recalls.

Knowing that her baby needed protein to grow, Valerie forced herself to eat as much meat as she could tolerate, even though it sat in her stomach and made her feel nauseated. "I worried that I wouldn't get enough protein otherwise," she says.

Valerie's uneasy relationship with meat continued through her next two pregnancies with daughters Zoe, now age 16, and Raven, age 12. Still, she never added more than 35 pounds to her 5-foot-5 frame with any of the kids. And each time, she lost the weight relatively quickly and resumed eating red meat without a problem.

Ironically, as Valerie's daughters got older, *they* began expressing a dislike for red meat. "They just refused to eat it," Valerie says. "Finally, my husband and I said, 'Well, we'll try being vegetarians for a month.' We never went back."

By the time Valerie became pregnant with her fourth child, she was a full-fledged vegetarian. She got her protein not from meat but from soy and dairy products, among other foods. "Making sure that I got enough protein helped me to be more aware of my food choices and eating habits," she says.

Valerie gained just 25 pounds before giving birth to daughter Mariah in October 1991. She credits a combination of vegetarian eating and breastfeeding with helping her to lose the extra weight.

Now age 44, Valerie is maintaining her weight at 129, just 9 pounds more than she weighed before she had her first child. She's convinced that her vegetarian lifestyle has played a huge part in keeping her fit and healthy for all these years.

WINNING ACTION

Expand your protein repertoire. No question about it: You need protein for your baby's healthy development. Red meat is among the best sources, because it's complete. In other words, it contains all nine essential amino acids. Unfortunately, it's also high in unhealthy saturated fat, which can contribute to unwanted weight gain.

Even if you don't want to give up red meat completely, consider incorporating some nonmeat protein sources into your diet. Low-fat dairy products and eggs are excellent choices, because they're complete proteins. Plant foods such as grains and beans are incomplete proteins, but you can make them complete by eating them in the right combinations.

HEALTH SCARE HAS HER
EATING BETTER THAN EVER

Melissa Baker had always considered herself a healthful eater. But when she became pregnant with twins, she redoubled her efforts to feed her body right. Even that wasn't enough to protect her from gestational diabetes, diagnosed between her sixth and seventh months. Learning to eat more often helped her not only to overcome the disease but also to lose 60 postpregnancy pounds.

A 31-year-old secretary from Whitehall, Pennsylvania, Melissa had struggled with an extra 10 to 15 pounds all of her life. So when she found out that she was going to have not one baby but two, she had reason to be concerned that she might end up with unwanted postpregnancy pounds. "I established better eating habits right away," she says. "I ate more fruits and vegetables, cut back on desserts, and gave up caffeine."

Melissa intended to continue her exercise routine as well. But eventually, she felt too exhausted to go to aerobics class. "Sometimes doctors advise pregnant women to cut back on their workouts, but that wasn't the case with me," she recalls. "I stopped on my own because I was just so tired."

Then a routine blood test between her 24th and 28th weeks of pregnancy revealed that Melissa had gestational diabetes. "I didn't want to endanger my babies another moment," she says. "I gathered as much information as I could, and I met with a nutritionist to find out what I could do to control the disease."

Though relatively rare, affecting only about 4 percent of pregnant women in the United States, gestational diabetes can have serious consequences for both mother and baby. Melissa was relieved to learn that she could control her condition through a combination of insulin injections and dietary changes. She didn't expect that she'd be eating as often as six times a day.

As her nutritionist explained, eating smaller meals more often would help Melissa keep her blood sugar on an even keel. "Instead of three big meals a day, it was more like six healthy snacks of mostly high-protein, low-fat, low-sodium foods," she explains.

This new way of eating not only helped control Melissa's blood sugar levels but also reined in her prenatal cravings. By the time she gave birth to daughters, Brianna and Brooke, in August 1999, she had added a healthy 60 pounds to her 5-foot-6 frame. "My doctor had told me not to worry about the weight gain, as long as I was getting proper nutrition," she says.

Within a week of the twins' arrival, Melissa's gestational diabetes was gone. Still, she stuck with her six-small-meals-a-day plan. "Nursing made me really hungry, so eating six times a day helped to control my appetite," she says. "When I'd get up in the middle of the night to feed the girls, I'd have something myself, like graham crackers and milk or an apple and a piece of cheese. Between that and nursing, the baby fat came off amazingly fast."

In fact, within 3 months, Melissa was back to her prepregnancy weight of 150 pounds. "Being pregnant and developing gestational diabetes taught me a lot about my body and how to take care of it," she says. "While I've gone back to three meals a day, I'm eating better than I have in my entire life."

WINNING ACTION

Eat smaller meals more often. *Even if you don't have gestational diabetes, you can benefit from dividing your standard three squares into five or six snack-size meals. As Melissa discovered, eating more frequently through-*

out the day helps keep cravings in check. What's more, it prevents you from taking in too many calories in one sitting—which is important, since your body can process only a certain number of calories at a time.

Note: If you've been diagnosed with gestational diabetes, don't make changes in your treatment plan without consulting your physician. She knows your situation best and can offer advice tailored to your unique nutritional and medical needs.

PRENATAL POOL TIME KEPT HER FIT

After working hard to take off the 19 pounds she had gained since college, Angela Van Meter was determined to stay in shape through her first pregnancy. But even she never expected to find herself in the delivery room just hours after exercising.

Angela, a 26-year-old legal assistant from Petersburg, West Virginia, first took up aqua aerobics and step aerobics to get her healthy lifestyle back on track. She had stayed active through high school and college, but once she entered the "real world," her fitness routine derailed. "I'd eat cake or doughnuts for breakfast and whatever I wanted for lunch," she recalls. "Then I'd go home and sit."

Over a period of 1½ years, Angela added 25 pounds to her 5-foot-3, 120-pound frame. "I felt my clothes getting tighter," she says. "But I lacked the motivation to do anything about it."

That changed when some of Angela's relatives who had weight problems themselves developed high cholesterol and high blood pressure. "I realized that I might be putting myself at risk unless I took steps to control my weight," she explains.

At first, Angela concentrated on reducing her fat intake. She also started walking on her lunch break at work. Later, feeling that she needed more of a challenge, she added aqua aerobics and step aerobics to her fitness routine. Between eating better and exercising regularly, Angela slimmed down to 126 pounds over the course of 1½ years. She maintained her weight until February 1999, when she found out that she was pregnant.

Angela admits that her eating habits started to slip fairly early in her pregnancy. "Because I was going to get big anyway, I gave myself the green light to eat what I wanted," she explains.

To compensate, Angela promised herself that she would continue working out as long as she could. Aqua aerobics turned out to be the perfect activity for this mom-to-be. "It not only kept me fit, it reduced my stress and helped me to sleep," she says. "It made me feel wonderful overall."

In fact, she was so enthusiastic about aqua aerobics that she earned her certification as an instructor while she was pregnant (with her doctor's approval, of course). "I had taken classes for so long that I figured becoming an instructor would give me a new perspective on the workouts," Angela explains. She received her certification just a month before delivering her baby.

Then one evening in November 1999, Angela worked out as usual. Around 9 o'clock, she went into labor. Her baby girl, Kerri, arrived 11 hours later.

Over the course of her pregnancy, Angela gained 46 pounds. She was eager to get back to her prepregnancy weight—but like most new moms, she had trouble finding time for exercise. So she and her husband compromised: Two nights a week, he stays home with the baby while she goes to her aqua aerobics class. She does the same for him. They also invested in a treadmill, which Angela uses after putting the baby to bed.

With her workouts back in full swing, Angela lost 34 pounds in 9 months. She's just 12 pounds shy of her prepregnancy weight—and confident that aqua aerobics will help her reach her goal.

WINNING ACTION

Move your prenatal workouts into the pool. *Aqua aerobics is one of the best forms of exercise for moms-to-be. It provides an excellent cardiovascular workout, with less risk of injury to knees and ankles. The water itself can provide great relief to women who are experiencing back pain. Many health clubs and YM/YWCAs offer classes tailored to pregnant women. Be sure to get your physician's okay before signing up.*

SHE'S POISED TO BECOME A WEIGHT-LOSS CHAMPION

Julie White is an odds-on favorite to clear the bar that sometimes separates new moms from their prepregnancy weights. The former Canadian Olympic high jumper is a lifelong devotee of healthy eating and consistent exercise. Now she's using the same discipline that made her a world-class athlete to ensure a healthy pregnancy and a speedy return to her prepregnancy physique.

After so many years of training for competition, Julie's commitment to fitness has become second nature. "I've been exercising my whole life," explains the 40-year-old Emmaus, Pennsylvania, resident. "I'm fortunate in that I've never had to diet." Indeed, when she became pregnant, she was a trim 5 feet 10 and 147 pounds.

Julie wanted to stay active, but she understood that the fitness regimen of an athlete—even a former athlete—might not pass muster for a mom-to-be. With her doctor's guidance, she made some modifications in her routine. "Through 8½ months, I was working out 4 days a week," she says. "That included 30 minutes on the stairclimber, plus weight training and stretching."

That certainly seems like a solid, even demanding, prenatal exercise program. But according to Julie, it wasn't nearly as intense as her usual regimen. "Since I finished competing, I've been running as my primary fitness activity," she says. "Before I became pregnant, I'd run for 30 to 90 minutes, usually 4 days a week."

As much as she enjoys exercising, Julie still has days when she struggles with motivation. "Even after all the years of training, getting excited about a workout can be a challenge," she says. "It's much easier to talk yourself out of exercising than to talk yourself into it. You need lots of discipline to persevere. I just keep reminding myself that if I exercise, I'll feel better afterward."

Discipline has also enabled Julie to make some minor but necessary adjustments in her dietary habits. "I used to drink a lot of diet Coke, but I've successfully cut out all caffeine and carbonated beverages," she says. "And except for the occasional handful of nacho chips, I've given up salty snacks as well."

Now in her ninth month, Julie has gained 33 pounds, which is considered healthy for someone her height. "I'm planning on breastfeeding, so I'll need to continue eating healthfully after I deliver," she says. "And I'd like to resume exercising as soon as possible." Sounds like Julie is destined to become a postpartum weight-loss winner!

WINNING ACTION

Make your healthy habits even better for you and baby.
If you were eating nutritiously and exercising regularly when you conceived, you have a great head start on a healthy pregnancy. Just bear in mind that you may need to make some adjustments as your pregnancy progresses and the demands on your body increase. Now is not the time to cut calories or rev up your fitness routine in an effort to control your prenatal weight gain. In fact, your doctor may advise you to do just the opposite. He can help you tweak your current eating and exercise habits to keep you fit and support your growing baby.

THIS MOM LEARNED TO LISTEN TO HER BODY

Long before she thought about becoming pregnant, Erin Pavlina was struggling with her weight. The Los Angeles resident adopted a vegan diet in an effort to clean up her eating habits and slim down. She didn't realize that veganism, which involves swearing off all animal products, has unhealthy temptations of its own.

Erin, who's now 31, laughs at the irony of describing herself as a formerly unhealthy vegan. "I used to eat lots of frozen vegan entrées for dinner," she says. "And I'm still trying to cut back on vegan junk food. You'd be surprised at how many of these products exist—even vegan doughnuts and vegan cookies."

Because the foods were vegan, Erin figured that she could eat as much as she wanted. In hindsight, she realizes that between her food choices and her portion sizes, she probably kept herself from slimming down.

Erin, who's 5 feet 9, weighed in at 187 pounds when she became pregnant in 1999. Concerned about her baby's nutrition, she strove for better food choices. She made sure to get enough lean protein by munching on lentils, chickpeas, cashews, and peas. She increased her calcium intake by drinking lots of fortified orange juice. She got more vitamin B_{12} by mixing nutritional yeast flakes into her food. "Instead of frozen entrées, I began preparing lots of fresh, low-fat, low-salt foods," she says.

Even with healthier foods on her plate, Erin knew that she had to watch her portion sizes. Taking in too many calories, no matter where they came from, would certainly make her gain too many pounds. She resolved to pay more attention to her body, feeding it only when she felt hungry and stopping when she felt satisfied. "A lot of women see pregnancy as a license to go crazy and eat as much as they want," she says. "I know better."

Because of her commitment to eating smarter, Erin held her prenatal weight gain to a healthy 20 pounds. She lost all of those pounds—plus 10 more—soon after giving birth to daughter Emily in February 2000. She has been holding steady at 177 ever since.

While she's thrilled to be below her prepregnancy weight, Erin would like to take off another 20 pounds. Her postpartum weight-loss success has her off to a good start. "Once you're headed in a positive direction, you don't want to lose any ground," she says.

WINNING ACTION

Eat when you're hungry; stop when you're satisfied. *Yes, you do need more calories during pregnancy—but perhaps not as many as you think. In fact, experts recom-*

mend only 200 to 300 extra calories per day during your second and third trimesters.

Your body will let you know when it needs food and when it has had enough. Pay attention for these signals. They'll help prevent episodes of overeating that can make you gain more than just baby fat.

PRENATAL ILLNESS CHANGES HER LIFE FOR THE BETTER

In 1994, while in her fifth month of pregnancy with her first child, Ellen Navitsky found out that she had gestational diabetes. At the time, the news was devastating. But looking back now, Ellen realizes that her diagnosis may have been a blessing in disguise. It forced her to make changes in her eating habits that controlled not only the disease but also her pregnancy weight gain.

Ellen had always tried to take good care of herself, eating healthfully and exercising regularly. At 5 feet 2 and 115 pounds, she seemed the picture of health—not a candidate for gestational diabetes. But diabetes runs in her family. "My grandmother has it, and so does my dad," says the 29-year-old Allentown, Pennsylvania, resident. "For some reason, I never thought of myself as being at risk."

As her doctor explained, Ellen likely developed gestational diabetes in part because of her family history, in part because she had taken the drug terbutaline (Brethine), which had been prescribed to prevent premature labor. Her doctor also said that she could control the disease by following a balanced diet with less refined sugar and more protein and fiber.

At first, Ellen struggled to deal with her diagnosis. "I cried every day when I had to test my blood," she recalls. "To me, that was worse than morning sickness." The dietary changes were tough, too, mostly because of Ellen's preference for carbohydrates. "I was accustomed to eating a bowl of cereal for breakfast and yogurt for lunch," she explains. "But that would make my blood sugar shoot through the roof."

With help from a nutritionist, Ellen learned that she could enjoy her favorite foods within the dietary guidelines for gestational diabetes. For instance, if she ate an apple, which is a carbohydrate, she'd also have a piece of cheese for protein. Likewise, when she started her day with a bowl of whole grain, low-sugar breakfast cereal (a carbohydrate), she'd pair it with some all-natural peanut butter (a protein).

By eating the right combinations of foods, Ellen was able to control her gestational diabetes without insulin injections. She noticed something else, too. "Even before I was pregnant, I had an incredible sweet tooth. Those cravings stopped, probably because my blood sugar was under control," she says. "Also, the protein seemed to fill me up, so I didn't eat as much."

Had she not been required to change her eating habits because of her gestational diabetes, Ellen might have gained a lot more weight through her pregnancy. Instead, she added just 30 pounds before giving birth to son Evan in January 1994. She started losing the weight almost immediately and was back to 115 about a year later. Even better, she showed no signs of diabetes just 2 months after her delivery.

When she became pregnant again in August 1998, Ellen had her healthy prenatal lifestyle down pat. She followed the same diet from her first pregnancy. She also adopted a fitness routine, doing lots of walking and bicycling as well as some light strength training.

(During her first pregnancy, her exercise was limited to walking, because of the risk of premature labor.) Once again, she held her pregnancy weight gain to 30 pounds, all of which disappeared within a year of daughter Olivia's arrival in May 1999.

As happy as Ellen is that she's back to her prepregnancy weight of 115 pounds, she's even more excited that she came through her second pregnancy without a hint of gestational diabetes. "It probably would have recurred had I not been more conscientious about my eating habits," she says. "Now I have a fighting chance to defy my family history and remain diabetes-free for the rest of my life."

WINNING ACTION

Control your cravings by pairing carbs and protein.
Cravings for sweets and other carbohydrates are sometimes fueled by a blood sugar imbalance. In moms-to-be, they can signal the onset of gestational diabetes. Even if you don't have the disease, you may be able to short-circuit cravings by pairing high-carbohydrate foods with a little bit of protein, such as crackers with peanut butter, an apple with cheese—even cookies with milk. The combination keeps your blood sugar in check, so you're less likely to binge and better able to maintain your pregnancy weight gain within a healthy range.

Note: If you've been diagnosed with gestational diabetes, don't make changes in your treatment plan without consulting your physician. He knows your situation best and can offer advice tailored to your unique nutritional and medical needs.

TEACHER LEARNS LESSON ABOUT THE VALUE OF PRENATAL FITNESS

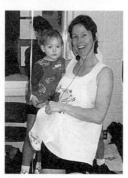

2 months before delivery

Susan Walker loves aerobics. She's so passionate about it that even pregnancy couldn't keep her away from her classes.

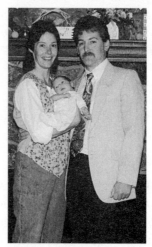

2 weeks after delivery

How could it? After all, she's the instructor.

Spend time with this 37-year-old mother of two from Monument, Colorado, and you'll quickly discover that fitness is a focal point of her life. "I've always enjoyed exercising," she says. "I like to keep myself in good shape." Her enthusiasm drove her decision to teach aerobics, which she has been doing for more than 10 years.

When Susan became pregnant with her oldest daughter, Ashley, in 1996, she saw no reason to change her routine. She felt fine, and she was having a ball. So with her doctor's approval, she continued teaching three or four classes a week all the way through her pregnancy. In fact, she had her last class just 4 days before she went into labor. "My students kept asking me if I was going to have my baby during class," she laughs.

Because she stayed active for the duration of her pregnancy, Susan added just 26 pounds to her 5-foot-6½ frame before Ashley's arrival in March 1997. Shortly after her delivery, she began walking regularly, and within a month, she slimmed down to 122 pounds, her prepregnancy weight. Four months postpartum, she was teaching aerobics classes again.

Just one year later, Susan became pregnant with her youngest daughter, Allison. She didn't push herself as hard this time around. "I was listening to my body," she explains. "I had days when I felt too tired to exercise, so I didn't." But she did teach three or four aerobics classes a week until her seventh month. That was enough to keep her prenatal weight gain to 27 pounds. She lost all of that baby fat soon after giving birth to Allison in May 1998.

Susan's pregnancies were such positive experiences that they inspired her to help other moms-to-be. Since earning her certification as a prenatal and postnatal fitness instructor, she designs workouts for women to follow during and after their pregnancies.

"I hear so many women say, 'I can't work out anymore—I'm pregnant,'" Susan says. "That's just not true. You can likely keep on doing what you're doing, as long as you enjoy it and your doctor approves it." She's living proof!

WINNING ACTION

Choose an activity that moves you. *Mustering the motivation to exercise isn't always easy. It can be downright daunting if you don't enjoy what you're doing. On the other hand, if you can identify an activity that brings you pleasure, you may find slipping on your workout clothes* *that much easier. Most experts recommend low-impact exercise—walking, stationary cycling, swimming, low-impact aerobics—for moms-to-be. But these aren't your only options. Ask your doctor for suggestions. Or check out your local health club or YM/YWCA for fitness classes tailored to moms-to-be.*

SHE'S PRIMING HER BODY FOR A WEIGHT-LOSS ENCORE

Gena Johnson has already won one battle with baby fat. But she's not resting on her laurels. Now expecting her second child, she's doing everything that she can to guarantee a repeat performance of a healthy pregnancy, a healthy baby, and a healthy postpregnancy weight loss.

For Gena, eating well and exercising regularly are a way of life. Her sensible habits helped her immensely when she became pregnant for the first time. "I ate lots of low-fat dishes—chicken, fish, some salads, lots of fruit," recalls the 35-year-old Waldorf, Maryland, resident. "Plus, I drank between 72 and 96 ounces of water a day, along with three servings of fat-free milk."

That's not to say that Gena didn't bend her nutrition rules. "I indulged my cravings with an occasional visit to Subway or Burger King," she admits. But the extra fat and calories hardly stood a chance: She also worked out almost every day, using indoor exercise machines, walking, and lifting weights.

Needless to say, Gena's commitment to staying fit paid off. She added just 27½ pounds to her 5-foot-4½, 115-pound body—an appropriate prenatal gain for someone her size. She gave birth to her son, Justin, in August 1999, and within 8 weeks, she had lost all of the baby fat—plus 2 extra pounds for good measure. She maintained her weight at 113 before becoming pregnant again.

Even with her previous weight-loss success, Gena is being just as diligent in her second pregnancy as in her first. She's not taking for granted that the pounds will come off easily. "I've already noticed that I'm having a harder time eating healthfully," she confesses. "I've done a lot of peanut butter and jelly sandwiches and a lot more fast food." She's faring better with her fitness routine, following the same one as before. Through 33½ weeks, she has put on 24 pounds.

As much as she wants to control her prenatal weight gain, Gena is being careful not to create unrealistic expectations for herself. She thinks that other moms-to-be should exercise the same caution. "Rushing to get rid of the baby fat only frustrates you, and it can hurt your body," she explains. "Even once you've lost the weight, you're going to need time to regain your prepregnancy figure." Good advice, from someone who has won the fat war once—and who is giving herself the best chance to do it again.

WINNING ACTION

Learn from past success—but don't assume that you'll repeat it. If you've lost postpregnancy pounds once, you may be tempted to relax your healthy habits this time around. While prior success certainly increases your chances of a repeat performance, it doesn't ensure one. After all, every pregnancy is unique. You may be confronted with different cravings, for example, or you may develop a medical condition that disrupts your fitness routine. Your best bet is to start with the strategies that worked before and make adjustments as necessary.

PREGNANCY TAMED HER TASTE FOR CHOCOLATE

Kathy Suder clearly remembers celebrating the news of her first pregnancy some 14 years ago. She did what any self-described chocolate addict might do: She went to a restaurant and ordered the biggest chocolate milkshake on the menu. It tasted so good that she promptly ordered another one.

Afterward, her sweet tooth was satisfied, but her conscience was not. "I thought that if I continued bingeing like that, I'd not only gain too much weight, but I might also compromise my baby's growth," explains Kathy, a 42-year-old Fort Worth, Texas, native. "I also realized that while I had a difficult time just bypassing sweets for my own health, I could do anything for my baby's health."

This was quite a revelation for someone who often joked that chocolate coursed through her veins. "You could have put me on an IV and loaded it with Hershey's Kisses!" she says.

Not wanting to jeopardize her baby for the sake of her sweet tooth, Kathy took action: She gave up chocolate, desserts, and sugary drinks—cold turkey. "I also avoided anything with artificial sweetener," she notes. Whenever she felt the urge to indulge, she'd just think about her growing baby to strengthen her willpower.

Kathy kept her diet healthy by eating plenty of fruits, vegetables, low-fat cheeses, and pasta dishes. To satisfy her cravings for meat, she treated herself to a cheeseburger each morning—a departure from her usual vegetarian eating habits.

Kathy's commitment to a sugar-free prenatal diet yielded sweet rewards. She gained just 16 pounds through her first pregnancy—ideal for her 5-foot-2, 120-pound body. "I suspect that giving up sugar helped me in other ways as well," she says. "I didn't have morning sickness at all. I felt wonderful the entire time."

In fact, Kathy felt so wonderful while carrying her firstborn, daughter Morgan, that she decided to give up sugar during her second and third pregnancies as well. She gained 32 pounds with son Jason, now age 12, and 25 pounds with Ryan, now 7. She lost the weight after each delivery, once she stopped breastfeeding. In the years since, she has slimmed down even more.

As her children have gotten older, Kathy's commitment to healthy eating has only grown stronger. She still enjoys chocolate, along with other sweets, but she doesn't crave it like she used to. "I allow myself an occasional treat," she says. "That's enough to satisfy my sweet tooth." And to preserve her trim figure: At 106 pounds, she's in the best shape of her life.

W I N N I N G   A C T I O N

Corral your chocolate cravings. *Research has shown that chocolate contains the same heart-protective compounds as red wine. But it has little else going for it in terms of nutrition, except plenty of calories and saturated fat. High intakes of sugar and fat not only contribute to weight gain but also may increase the risk of a serious prenatal condition called preeclampsia.*

You don't need to give up sweets completely. On the other hand, you don't want them to be a fixture in your prenatal diet. When you get a craving for something chocolatey or sugary, try eating a piece of fresh fruit. That may be enough to satisfy you. If you still want chocolate, choose something low-fat or fat-free, perhaps a cup of cocoa made with 1% milk or a frozen fudge bar.

YOGA PRIMED HER BODY AND MIND FOR BABY

Ask new mom Lynne Brolly how she stayed in shape during her pregnancy, and she'll likely give much of the credit to yoga. She's convinced that daily yoga sessions prepared her mentally and physically for childbirth—and kept away excess postpregnancy pounds.

Lynne, a first-time mom, got word that she was expecting in November 1999. At the time, she had been a yoga devotee for some 13 years. "When I found out that I was pregnant, there was no question that I would continue to practice yoga," explains the 37-year-old administrative assistant from Mertztown, Pennsylvania. "It had been a part of my life for so long."

Lynne did have to make some adjustments to her routine, however. She and her husband went from between 1 and 2 hours of practice to just ½ hour before heading to work each morning. She continued to take three yoga classes a week and teach another. Her doctor approved of Lynne's rigorous schedule, though she did advise Lynne to avoid certain postures, for her safety and her baby's.

Lynne's prenatal care also included some changes to her diet. A vegetarian for almost 20 years, she made a point of eating more dairy products, peanut butter, beans, and soy protein to support her growing baby. Because of her diligence and commitment to a healthy pregnancy, she added only 30 pounds to her 5-foot-6, 145-pound frame before delivering son Hugh in August 2000.

Looking back, Lynne can't help marveling at how yoga kept her fit through her pregnancy. And the meditations she learned through yoga helped her to relax and relieve prepregnancy tension. "Yoga helped me to be more aware of the changes my body was going through and to make peace with them," she explains. "Because I was attuned to what was happening to me physically, I understood that my body was going to get back to normal eventually."

Since having her baby, Lynne has resumed the running and walking workouts that helped to keep her slim and in shape before her pregnancy. But that doesn't mean she's given up her first love, yoga. On the contrary, "I can't go a day without it!" she says.

WINNING ACTION

Practice yoga to prepare your body for childbirth. *Many gyms offer prenatal yoga classes, perfect for the woman who wants a safe, non-impact activity to manage her pregnancy weight gain. Some doctors feel that regular yoga practice can also make for an easier delivery.*

Be sure to look for a certified yoga instructor who understands the special needs of moms-to-be. And get the approval of your doctor before taking up yoga or any new exercise routine.

CARRYING TWINS DOUBLES HER DETERMINATION

She has already given birth to three children, and each time she has lost the postpregnancy pounds. Now Cristine Boedecker faces a bigger challenge: She's expecting twins! Her goal is to gain enough weight to nourish her growing babies, but not so much that she has lots to lose once the twins arrive.

Cristine's current brood includes adopted daughter Alisha, 12; son Blake, 9; and daughters Michaela, 7, and Kiley, 5. During each of her previous pregnancies, she controlled her weight gain with a combination of healthful eating habits and doctor-approved exercise. But now that she's carrying twins, her doctor has cautioned her to cut back on some of the high-impact activities that she enjoys.

"Before being put on semi–bed rest at 20 weeks, I continued my usual fitness routine—walking, running, high-impact aerobics, and light strength training to tone my muscles," says the 29-year-old Owatonna, Minnesota, resident. "It not only kept me in shape, it also was a great stress reliever."

Cristine, who stands 5 feet 3, weighed 115 pounds at the start of her pregnancy. According to the experts, a woman her size who's expecting twins should put on between 35 and 45 pounds. That's more than the 25 to 30 pounds she gained—and lost—in each of her previous pregnancies.

So now Cristine finds herself in the unusual, and perhaps slightly enviable, position of having to eat *more* than she did before. "This is week 26, and I've gained 13 pounds," she notes. "I've almost doubled my normal food intake to get adequate nutrition for my babies and me."

Even with the higher caloric demands of carrying twins, Cristine strives to make food choices that will help her stay healthy now and take off the baby fat later. "I limit sweets, which isn't hard because I don't have a sweet tooth," she says. "I still wouldn't eat a doughnut if you put one in front of me." Likewise, she shuns junk food and anything fried.

Cristine knows that she's going to gain more weight than in her previous pregnancies, but she isn't worried about slimming down. "After carrying two babies for 9 months and concentrating on their needs, I'm kind of looking forward to focusing on myself for a little while," she says. She relied on aerobics to help her take off the post-pregnancy pounds before, and she thinks she'll do the same again.

"It toned my muscles and made me feel stronger. It helped me lose the weight rather quickly," she says. "Besides, I enjoy it!"

W I N N I N G   A C T I O N

Expect twins to change the rules of prenatal weight management. *When you're carrying twins, your body's caloric needs increase proportionately, and you gain more than you would with one baby. But only about 10 pounds more, according to the experts. So while you may need to increase your food intake, you must be careful not to overeat or to load up on empty calories. Packing on too many pounds can increase your risk of complications, including cesarean delivery.*

FROM BOUNCING BALLS TO A BOUNCING BABY BOY

For 11 years, basketball played a major role in Jaime Berg Moomau's life. During that time, she learned a lot about training, conditioning, and taking care of her body. Her knowledge would come in handy as she prepared for the physical demands of pregnancy and childbirth. It would also help her score a victory over those post-pregnancy pounds.

Jaime, a gifted athlete, has been passionate about sports for as long as she can remember. She started playing basketball in third grade and continued through her first year of college. "Back then, I didn't need an exercise routine, because practice kept me so busy," recalls the 24-year-old Maysville, West Virginia, resident. "But when

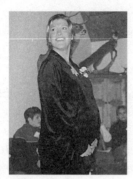

2 weeks before delivery

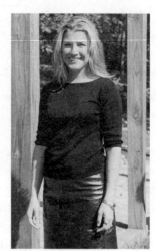

6½ months after delivery

I stopped playing, I figured that I'd have to find some other way to stay in shape."

Jaime continued walking, running, and strength training—the same activities that had kept her in peak condition for basketball. Eventually, she joined a gym, where she used the stairclimber and treadmill, in addition to lifting weights. Jaime's efforts paid off: At 5 feet 7½ and 144 pounds, she was in great shape when she became pregnant in June 1999.

The prospect of motherhood could have persuaded Jaime to pack up her workout clothes and take a break for the next 9 months. Instead, it gave her even more reason to continue her training. "From the start of my pregnancy, my primary goal was to stay healthy, for me and for my baby," she explains. "I also wanted to control the amount of weight that I gained, so I didn't have to lose a lot afterward. Besides, many of the women at the gym told me that they had an easy labor, and they attributed it to exercise."

Like many moms-to-be, Jaime had to make some adjustments in her fitness program to accommodate her baby. She walked about

4 miles three times a week and took aqua aerobics classes two times a week. She continued strength training to maintain muscle tone. "I also made some changes in my diet," she says. "I tried to make food choices with my baby in mind."

Between eating nutritiously and exercising almost daily, Jaime held her prenatal weight gain to a healthy 29 pounds. And every one of those pounds came off within 3 months of son Jackson's arrival in February 2000. "Because of some problems during labor, I had to undergo an emergency cesarean section," she says. "But I think that being in shape helped me to quickly recover from the surgery.

"During my pregnancy, I had moments when I'd look in the mirror and wonder whether those extra pounds would ever disappear," Jaime adds. "But now I realize that exercising is the best thing that I could have done. I'm healthy—and more important, my son is healthy."

WINNING ACTION

View prenatal exercise as training for an athletic event.
Many women have likened giving birth to running a marathon: It's physically demanding, and it can last for hours. That's why training and conditioning are just as important for moms-to-be as for athletes. Of course, you don't want to overdo, which can harm you and your baby. But even moderate exercise can build your strength and stamina. And that not only makes giving birth easier, it also makes losing those postpregnancy pounds easier.

PREGNANCY JUMP-STARTS HER WEIGHT-LOSS EFFORTS

Overweight for most of her life, Polly Smith worried about getting even heavier when she became pregnant for the first time. Now she weighs less than before she had her son, Jackson—and her success in taking off those postpregnancy pounds has inspired her to believe that she can achieve even greater weight-loss success.

Polly distinctly remembers when her weight problems began. "Puberty came early for me," recalls the 32-year-old Vicksburg, Mississippi, resident. "I was in third grade when I got my first bra. My weight started changing at about the same time."

Both of Polly's parents battled weight problems over the years, which led Polly to believe that she has some genetic predisposition to obesity. But she also puts some of the blame for her weight gain on her own inattentiveness to her eating and exercise habits. When she became pregnant in March 1998, she was carrying 266 pounds on her 5-foot-8 frame.

Although the odds seemed stacked against her, Polly was determined not to let her prenatal weight gain spin out of control. "I knew that I would have to eat better," she says. "I drank a lot of water, which helped control my appetite. I cut back on junk food, especially candy and other sweets. I tried to make good food choices for my baby and me."

Because of these changes, Polly actually lost some weight early in her pregnancy. By the time she gave birth to Jackson in December 1998, she had gained just 21 pounds—an amount that pleased both her and her doctor.

Polly continued to eat healthfully while nursing her son. "Actually, I wasn't all that hungry then," she says. "When I did eat, I had to be really careful because my son had reflux. The slightest change in my diet would upset his stomach."

Between breastfeeding and making smart food choices, Polly lost the 21 postpregnancy pounds—plus 14 more—within 4 weeks of Jackson's arrival. She has been holding steady at 252 pounds ever since. "I'm eating better now than I did before I got pregnant," she says. "And my son started walking at 9½ months, so I'm getting lots of exercise just chasing after him!"

Now that she has seen what she's capable of accomplishing, Polly is set to tackle an even loftier goal. "Honestly, I've never been all that weight-conscious, but I'd like to get down to 200, if not lower," she says. "I feel good, but I'd love to lose more. Lots more!"

WINNING ACTION

Use your pregnancy as a springboard to achieving even greater weight-loss success. *If you were overweight when you became pregnant, you might be extra-anxious about putting on those pregnancy pounds—and getting rid of them afterward. Instead, look at the next 9 months as an opportunity to change your lifestyle for the better. Eating more healthfully and exercising regularly will benefit you as well as your baby. And who knows? Your success at slimming down after pregnancy just might give you incentive to pursue an even bigger weight-loss goal.*

Lose the Postpartum Pouch

FIT BEFORE HER PREGNANCY, SHE'LL BE FIT AGAIN

Giving birth is a workout in itself. Most new moms welcome a little rest and relaxation after the extraordinary physical demands of labor and delivery. Not Catherine Bowen Brophy. After delivering her first child, she couldn't wait to resume her fitness routine. It had kept her in shape before, so it would certainly help her slim down to her prepregnancy weight.

Catherine, a 33-year-old public relations professional, had been walking regularly for years. When her employer offered a beginner-level yoga class at its corporate fitness center, she added that to her exercise program. "I signed up because I thought yoga might be a good stress reliever—and it was," she explains. "But it also helped to trim and tone my body, which I hadn't expected."

Catherine enjoyed her yoga sessions so much that when she moved to Newport, Rhode Island, to start her own company, she searched for—and found—a yoga class that would allow her to continue developing her skills. She also continued her walking routine. "Newport is very scenic, so I can vary my routes," she says. "I walk to clients' offices, to nearby shops, to the beach, and, of course, to the famed mansions."

A short time after moving to Newport, Catherine learned that she was pregnant. "My doctor was very 'pro-yoga,' and he encouraged me to stay with it through my pregnancy," Catherine says. "I enrolled in a special prenatal yoga class that concentrated more on breathing, stretching, and visualization. It prepared me physically and mentally for the birthing process, and as a bonus, it helped control my prenatal weight gain."

In fact, the combination of once- or twice-weekly yoga practice and daily walks kept Catherine within 31 pounds of her prepregnancy weight. "I didn't need to make too many dietary changes, since I'm normally a healthy eater," she notes. When she delivered daughter Erin in May 2000, she was carrying 133 pounds on her petite 5-foot-2 frame.

Catherine was thrilled that her prenatal weight gain had stayed within a healthy range. But she wanted to lose the extra pounds as quickly as possible. So 2 to 3 weeks after having her baby, she eased back into her fitness routine.

She started out by walking 1½ miles every other day, often taking Erin along in a carrier. That alone was enough to take off 20 pounds in 9 weeks.

In retrospect, Catherine knows that staying active through her pregnancy has made slimming down afterward much easier. Because of her success so far, she's confident that she'll eventually return to her prepregnancy weight. The fitness routine that has kept her slim and shapely for many years will undoubtedly help her shed those last postpregnancy pounds.

WINNING ACTION

Pick up where you left off. *Most obstetricians recommend waiting at least 6 weeks after delivery before resuming strenuous physical activity. Before then, you may be able to do some low-intensity walking or other gentle exercise. Once you have your doctor's okay, you can gradually ease back into your fitness routine. If you don't have a regular program, work with your doctor or a fitness professional to develop one that not only whittles away the baby fat but also supports the postpartum healing process.*

HER WEIGHT-LOSS SUCCESS IS ALL IN HER HEAD

Sometimes just telling yourself that you can slim down helps to melt away those postpregnancy pounds. It certainly worked for Heather Lee. The 37-year-old Charlottesville, Virginia, resident repeats her own motivational mantras while working out. They've helped her to take off 42 pounds of baby fat so far.

Heather gave birth to daughter Teagan in September 1999. "I was glad that winter was on the way," she recalls. "I figured that I could conceal my body underneath baggy sweaters and pants." Normally 5-foot-3 and 109 pounds, she had gained about 45 pounds during her pregnancy. And the extra weight didn't come off as quickly as she had hoped.

Heather's plan to hide her body under bulky clothes was foiled when her family was invited to spend the holidays in Florida. "I panicked at the thought of donning a bathing suit," she says. "I made some feeble attempts at exercise, but the cold weather wiped out my motivation."

By the time the holidays rolled around, Heather hadn't lost so much as a pound. "I went to Florida, flabby and pale," she laughs. "Thank goodness nursing triggers the release of hormones that make a woman feel good. Otherwise, I might not have survived."

Heather's baby fat stuck around until spring, when her determination to slim down returned. "I felt really inspired by the weather and the approach of summer," she says. "I wanted to be ready for my 'unveiling' by the pool."

Four mornings a week, with her husband at home to watch the baby, Heather went out for a run—something she had done regularly before her pregnancy. She used affirmations to maintain her motivation during her workouts. "The affirmations grew out of my journaling, in which I'd write positive statements to boost my spirits," she explains. "When I started running, I just kept chanting these statements over and over again, to drown out any negative inner chatter. Some of my favorites were 'With every step, I get firmer and fitter,' 'My body gravitates toward fitness,' and 'I feel strong, healthy, and sexy!'"

Between running and repeating her affirmations—and with some help from a prudent eating plan that included balanced meals but no snacks—Heather finally started shedding her postpregnancy pounds. That made her feel more enthusiastic and upbeat each time she'd exercise. "Focusing on these positive statements for 45 minutes is an incredible experience," she says. "I'm totally convinced that they have a positive effect on my physiology. In some way, they seem to program my body to slim down more quickly."

Within 6 months, Heather lost all but 3 of her postpregnancy pounds, putting her within easy reach of her prepregnancy weight. "By bathing suit season, I still had some toning to do," she says, "but I felt confident about myself and my body." She intends to keep on running and chanting her motivational mantras until she gets there. "For me, running has become a moving meditation," she says. "It's powerful stuff!"

WINNING ACTION

Develop a mindset that fosters weight-loss success. *Time and again, studies have shown that the mind exerts a powerful, profound influence over the body. Just by believing that you can slim down, you may actually increase your chances of succeeding. That's why you should consider making affirmations part of your weight-loss plan. You can create your own empowering state-*

*ment, anything from a simple "I can do it" to a more de-
tailed recitation of the health benefits of taking off those
extra pounds. Then repeat it whenever you need to, as
often as you need to. Feel your self-confidence soar!*

FOR NO-SWEAT WEIGHT LOSS, JUST FOLLOW IN THIS MOM'S FOOTSTEPS

Lisa Gordon took a step-by-step approach to slimming down. Literally. The 30-year-old Pittsburgh resident found ingenious ways to
increase the number of steps in her daily routine. In the process, she
lost all 30 of her postpregnancy pounds.

Lisa has always been a firm believer in exercising and eating
right. But when she became pregnant in June 1999, she went from
working out two or three times a week to feeling too exhausted to
even go to the gym. On top of that, her healthy dietary habits gave
way to fast-food cravings. "I'd stop at McDonald's for a burger or
fish sandwich on my way home from work," she recalls. "My husband, David, would say to me, 'We're eating dinner in a half-hour.'
And I'd tell him, 'I can't wait. I'm hungry now.'"

Eating also helped Lisa fend off nausea. "I needed food in my
stomach at all times," she explains. "As soon as it was empty, I'd start
feeling sick."

In her first trimester alone, Lisa—who's 5 feet 6—went from
125 to 155 pounds. Her doctor cautioned that if she kept going at
that rate, she'd be overweight by her due date. Fortunately, that
didn't happen. Her cravings, and her excessive weight gain, ended

after her third month. She never put on more than those 30 pounds.

After giving birth to daughter Rachel by cesarean section in February 2000, Lisa took her baby fat off with minimal effort. But she knew that to keep it off, she'd have to stay active.

"For the first week or so after the C-section, I was supposed to keep walking to a minimum. So my husband moved Rachel's changing table downstairs," Lisa says. "Once I was able to go up steps again, I asked him to take the table back up to the nursery."

Lisa made at least 12 trips up and down the stairs each day—7 to 10 just to change Rachel's diapers, plus several more to put her down for naps and bedtime. "People kept asking me, 'Why don't you just change her on the couch?'" Lisa recalls. "They didn't understand that I had to do something to get moving."

Keeping the changing table on the second floor of her home was just one way in which Lisa added more steps to her daily routine. Three or four times a week, she headed out for a 45-minute walk with a neighbor. On inclement days, she loaded Rachel and the stroller into the car and drove to the nearest mall, where she did her walking. And when she went to the supermarket or drugstore, she parked as far away from the entrance as possible.

Thanks to all of that extra mileage, Lisa has managed to maintain her weight at 125 pounds since 3 months after giving birth. "It's just a few steps at a time," she says. "But over the course of a day, they really add up!"

WINNING ACTION

Slim down, one step at a time. With every extra step, you burn a few more calories. Over the course of a day, it can really make a difference. Think of ways in which you can increase your foot mileage. Lisa's decision to keep her *baby's changing table in the second-floor nursery is a great example. Other suggestions: When you're talking on the phone, pace around rather than sitting down. If you have a multi-story home, or if you work in an office building, use the bathroom on another floor. When you head to the mall, take a couple of laps to check out all of the sales before you start buying. You'll burn more calories—and maybe save a few bucks to boot.*

SHE LOVES TO LOSE

Leanne MacLeod knew that she had a good thing going. Within 6 weeks of delivering her first child, she lost *twice* the number of pounds that she had gained through her pregnancy. She wanted to lose even more. She felt that she owed it to her baby and, just as important, to herself.

Leanne and her husband very much wanted to become parents. So when the Toronto couple learned that Leanne was expecting, they were positively thrilled. Still, Leanne had some concerns about the pending weight gain. At 5 feet 3 and 155 pounds, "I didn't feel I had a major weight problem, but I knew that I would have been thinner if I had taken better care of my body," she says.

During her pregnancy, Leanne gained just 12 pounds—less than the 15 to 25 pounds recommended for a woman her size. "Low weight gain was normal for women in my family," Leanne explains. "I did a lot of walking while I was pregnant, too." Still, she was amazed at how quickly she slimmed down after son Kevin's arrival in December 1999. "When I weighed myself 5 days after Kevin was born, I had already lost 15 pounds," she recalls. "By my 6-week post-partum checkup, I had lost 25 pounds total."

Inspired by her unexpected slimming, Leanne was determined not only to keep off the weight but also to take off more. After 9 months of pregnancy, she had earned the right to pay a little extra attention to herself. "I chose to eat better and exercise more because I wanted to feel good," she explains. "When you do something for your own benefit, it really boosts your self-esteem."

Leanne didn't make any major changes in her eating habits, though she continued to be careful about her food choices. For exercise, her activity of choice was walking, with her son as her companion. Later, she began taking step aerobics at her community center once or twice a week. "My son and I will also be taking a swimming class together, which will help me shape up," she says.

Leanne, who is now 21, figures that she has to lose another 20 or so pounds to reach her own ideal weight of 110 to 115. "My husband and I would like to have another baby soon," she says. "I know that if I don't slim down now, I may have a harder time after my next pregnancy."

But rather than dwelling on what she still must accomplish, Leanne takes pride in how far she has come. "I love fitting into clothes in sizes that I never dreamed I'd be able to wear," she says. "And when someone compliments me on my appearance, I feel even better. I know that I'm doing right by taking care of myself."

WINNING ACTION

Put yourself first for a change. *As a mom, you may become so focused on your family's needs that you completely set aside your own. But by putting your fitness routine or your healthy eating habits on the back burner,* *you risk letting those pounds of baby fat become permanent. You do so much good for others that you <u>deserve</u> to do something good for yourself. And you shouldn't feel the least bit guilty about it. You might want to talk with your spouse about scheduling 30 minutes to an hour of "alone time" every day. He can watch the kids while you exercise, plan your meals for the week, or simply relax and unwind. Managing stress is just as important to your weight-loss efforts as burning calories.*

MIRROR IMAGE MADE HER WANT TO LOSE

As a single mother and full-time college student with a part-time job, Amanda Goetz had little time to worry about losing all of the 41 pounds she had gained while pregnant. That was okay with her. Except for an extra "pouch" across her midsection, she felt comfortable with her appearance.

Her accepting attitude began to change soon after her longtime boyfriend decided to end their relationship. "We didn't break up because I had gotten heavier," explains the 20-year-old Ann Arbor, Michigan, native. "But when it happened, I realized that I wasn't happy with myself. Comfortable, but not happy."

Amanda had lost some of the weight from her pregnancy within 2 months of giving birth to daughter Jacqueline. But most of it had hung around for 2 years.

"I realized that I had more or less settled on being heavier because I didn't feel any pressure to change," she says. "Once I was on my own again I had to admit that I wasn't satisfied with my appearance. The extra pounds had to go."

With so much already on her plate, Amanda still manages to squeeze exercise sessions into her daily routine. She practices figure skating every morning—she's a member of her university's skating team—and often uses her lunch hour to go to the university's gym. There, she takes Tae-Bo classes, uses the strength-training equipment, and occasionally does yoga. If she can't work out over lunch, she squeezes in some activity when she gets home. "My daughter likes to watch," she says with a smile.

Because she has always been fairly conscientious about her eating habits, Amanda hasn't made any major changes in her diet. "I don't like red meat, but I love pasta and salads," she says. "I make sure that my daughter eats well, too."

Once she decided to lose her remaining postpregnancy pounds, Amanda couldn't believe how quickly she saw results. She shed 25 pounds within 1½ months. Just 16 pounds more, and the 5-foot-4 Amanda will be down to 110, her prepregnancy weight.

Even though she has not quite reached her goal, Amanda loves the changes in her body so far. "I actually like looking at myself in the mirror," she says. "I can see that I've made progress. That extra weight around my midsection is practically gone!"

WINNING ACTION

Launch your postpartum weight-loss program when you feel ready. Once Amanda made up her mind to shed her postpregnancy pounds, she could commit herself to the fitness routine that would help her slim down, even though it meant carving more time out of her already hectic schedule. That desire is so important to weight-

loss success. It can be tough to muster when you're grappling with all of the other changes that accompany the arrival of a new family member. Give yourself the time you need. Allow other aspects of your life to settle down before launching a weight-loss program. You'll feel better about doing something good for yourself.

THIS MOM STANDS UP TO TEMPTATION

You might not think of a hospital as a dietary danger zone. Neither did Tracy Fleischman, who works in one. But while on leave after delivering her first child—daughter Amber, who's now 2—she realized just how much she ate on the job. She knew that had to change if she wanted to take off her postpregnancy pounds.

Before her pregnancy, Tracy—a 30-year-old Wheatfield, New York, resident—could eat pretty much what she wanted. It didn't seem to have any effect on her trim, 130-pound figure. "Often I'd have a big lunch in the cafeteria, or I'd go out with coworkers," she says. "For a snack, I'd buy candy in the gift shop."

Tracy didn't make any major changes in her eating habits while pregnant. But once she was at home taking care of her newborn daughter, she noticed that she was eating better. "I wasn't snacking as much," she recalls. "I had my three basic meals, and I didn't go back for seconds." She paid more attention to her food choices, too, replacing high-fat items like french fries and potato chips with more nutritious fruits and vegetables.

By trimming her snacks and eating more healthful meals, Tracy lost all 34 of her postpregnancy pounds, plus 3 extra, within 4 months. When she eventually returned to work, she made sure that her new and improved eating habits went along. She maintained her weight at 127 pounds until she became pregnant with her second child.

"I know that I can't eat anything I want anymore," Tracy says. "But that's okay, because I'm not missing the snacks and the high-fat foods. I'm doing what's best for my baby and me."

WINNING ACTION

Identify your dietary danger zones. *Proximity to food is an all-too-common weight-loss saboteur. You may find yourself eating whether or not you're hungry, simply because food is available. In Tracy's case, the danger zone was her workplace, where she could get anything she wanted, anytime she wanted. Fortunately, she corrected her eating habits before they turned her postpregnancy pounds into permanent baby fat. You may face temptation while shopping, running errands, or even puttering around at home. Do a mental run-through of your daily routine, homing in on situations that might jeopardize your postpartum weight-loss goals. Then think of ways to avoid eating in those situations, or at least to make more healthful food choices.*

EXERCISE COMES FIRST ON HER DAILY AGENDA

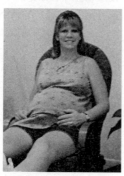

9 months pregnant

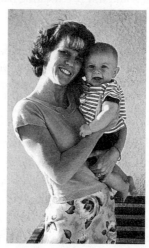

7 months after delivery

At 6:30 in the morning, while many of us are hitting the snooze alarm and snuggling under the covers to grab a few more minutes of shut-eye, 33-year-old Victoria Scuro is slipping on her workout clothes. Her early-morning exercise sessions have become a ritual since son Nikolas was born. They're the primary reason for this mom's 64-pound postpregnancy weight loss.

Considered high-risk by her doctors, Victoria had to keep her feet up for much of her pregnancy. Exercise was off-limits. With 9 months of cheese and chicken-nugget cravings and little physical activity, her 5-foot-6 physique grew from 135 pounds to 180.

After giving birth to Nikolas in October 1999, Victoria lost 20 pounds of baby fat right off the bat. But she remained well above her goal weight of 125.

Victoria knew that to shed the rest of her postpregnancy pounds, she'd need to resume her fitness program. She started out by putting Nikolas in his stroller and walking him around their Thousand Palms, California, neighborhood once or twice a day.

"I wanted to exercise more, but I just couldn't seem to get motivated," she explains. "Then I saw a photo of me that had been taken at Christmas. I was all hips! That gave me the push I needed. I went out and bought a Tae-Bo tape the next day."

Three mornings a week, Victoria did her video workout. "I'd lay out my exercise clothes the night before, and as soon as I'd get out of bed, I'd put them on," she says. She started with a beginner-level workout, learning all kinds of kicks, punches, and stretches. By May, she was ready to move on to a more advanced tape.

Exercising in the morning has enabled Victoria to avoid the distractions that might have otherwise derailed her fitness program. "At that hour, no one is going to call or knock on the door," she says. "If I put off my workout until my husband gets home from work, we'll eat dinner first—and then something will invariably come up."

Another advantage of Victoria's early-morning workouts is that even though her son is awake, he's content to entertain himself. "When Nikolas was an infant, he'd watch me from his swing or bouncy seat," she says. "When he started crawling, he'd sometimes come over and untie my shoes or hang onto my leg. But he'd usually give me that time."

Thanks to her A.M. exercise, Victoria reached her goal weight of 125 pounds just 5 months after giving birth to Nikolas. She has lost even more since then, and is now holding steady at 116. "Even my prepregnancy clothes are loose!" she says.

WINNING ACTION

Plan your workouts for first thing in the morning. *By exercising at the start of your day, you can avoid the distractions that so often disrupt even the best-laid fitness* *plans. You may need to roll out of bed earlier than usual—but after your workout, you'll have more energy to get through the rest of the day. Follow Victoria's lead and lay out your exercise clothes the night before, so you can slip them on as soon as you get up in the morning.*

50 POUNDS LIGHTER, SHE'S READY FOR HER CLOSE-UP

For a new mom who happens to work in the public eye, the pressure to slim down soon after delivery can be tremendous. No one knows that better than 35-year-old Connie Colla, a former news anchor for the NBC 10 morning news in Philadelphia.

During her pregnancy, Connie stayed fit by eating healthfully—"I craved fat-free hot dogs and cheese, of all things," she says—and by walking every other day. Her job kept her quite active, too. She added 35 pounds to her 5-foot-7 body before giving birth to daughter Sophia in November 1999.

As thrilled as Connie was to become a mother, she knew that she had to recapture her prepregnancy figure quickly. "I'm in a very competitive business, and appearance means a lot," she explains. "I just had to take off the weight."

Within 2 to 3 weeks, Connie started going to a gym, working out almost every day. At first, she focused her attention on aqua aerobics and low-impact aerobics. Once she felt a little stronger, she moved on to kickboxing.

While all of these activities helped trim and tone Connie's body, she noticed the most improvement once she began practicing Pilates (pronounced "pi-LAH-teez"). The brainchild of German fitness expert Joseph Pilates, it consists of a series of low-impact movements designed to build strength and flexibility. It has grown in popularity in recent years, especially among new moms, as it gently firms and sculpts their bodies after pregnancy.

After reading about Pilates in a magazine, Connie signed up for private lessons at her local gym. She enjoyed the exercises so much that she began doing them twice a week. She continued her routine once she returned to work, when Sophia was 2 months old.

"The Pilates exercises helped me regain muscle tone throughout my body," Connie says. And because they focused on strengthening her abdominal muscles and improving her posture, she appeared much slimmer, especially around her midsection.

Indeed, within 7 months of her daughter's arrival, Connie had lost her 35 postpregnancy pounds, plus 15 more. Now she's looking better than ever. And she's still practicing Pilates. "I like it because it's not strenuous, yet it tones my muscles and makes me look leaner," she says. "It has produced dramatic results for me."

WINNING ACTION

Shape your postpartum physique with Pilates. *Once a well-kept secret of the stars (including Sharon Stone, Madonna, and Julia Roberts), the Pilates method has gone mainstream. It's great for new moms (with a doctor's approval), because it provides a gentle workout, with no jerky, bouncy movements. And it targets the abdominal muscles, which are in urgent need of toning after pregnancy. While Pilates classes have become quite common, you may prefer personalized instruction, at* *least until you learn to do the exercises correctly. For a referral to a certified instructor in your area, call 800-PILATES (800-745-2837).*

FOR THIS MOM, WEIGHT LOSS IS A GROUP EFFORT

First-time mom Sharlene Tupas has no doubt that she'll lose her 35 postpregnancy pounds. After all, the 30-year-old from Silverdale, Washington, has her very own support team to help her do it.

Sharlene belongs to a close-knit group of women, all of whom are married to naval officers. For years, they have met regularly for coffee and conversation, along with other social activities. "We really enjoy each other's company, especially when our husbands are out at sea on assignment," she says.

That camaraderie was especially valuable to Sharlene after she gave birth to her son, Kyle, who's now 9 months old. The moms in the group had all sorts of good advice—not just about motherhood but also about weight loss. "I could ask them about almost anything," she says. "They had already been in the same situation, so they could offer really helpful pointers for my baby and me."

Because Sharlene was breastfeeding, she knew that she couldn't diet or engage in strenuous exercise. But the other moms suggested some healthy changes in her lifestyle. She gave up all sugary snacks and focused on eating more fruits and vegetables. "Staying away from sweets has been hard, but I just keep reminding myself that I need to do that if I want to slim down," she says. For the same reason, she also began walking around her neighborhood for about 40 minutes every day, except on weekends.

While Sharlene treasured the wisdom and experience of the

mothers in her group, she also drew inspiration from the non-moms. "They're very trim and fit, so they're also good role models for me," she says. "I want to look as great as they do."

Since delivering Kyle, Sharlene, who's 5 feet 9, has lost 25 of her 35 postpregnancy pounds. She'll need to stay committed to her healthy habits in order to shed the rest of her baby fat and reach 160, her prepregnancy weight. The other wives understand that. "They give me so much strength and support," she says. "They're going to make sure that I succeed."

W I N N I N G   A C T I O N

Learn from those who have been there before you.
When you were pregnant, you likely had lots of women, moms themselves, telling you what to do and what to expect. And you probably learned something from their experiences. Now that you've had your baby, you can tap into their knowledge again. Ask them what they did to lose their postpregnancy pounds and regain their prepregnancy figures. Of course, what worked for one woman won't necessarily produce the same results for you. But you can certainly experiment with their strategies to see which seem to help.

SHE HAS A PICTURE-PERFECT WEIGHT-LOSS PLAN

The day Karla Kiedinger took her firstborn child, Sarah, home from the hospital is a memorable one, though for a reason you may not expect. As thrilled as Karla was to be a mom, she was dismayed to discover that she still weighed 180 pounds—as much as she did during her pregnancy.

Before she became pregnant, the 34-year-old Lawrenceville, Georgia, resident had carried just 138 pounds on her 5-foot-4 frame. But the photos from her baby's homecoming day in September 1999 show a much heavier woman. "I literally couldn't stand the sight of myself," Karla says. "I was huge!"

Those photos became Karla's motivation for shedding her baby fat as quickly as possible. To help her succeed, she opted to go on the Slim-Fast plan, which uses meal-replacement shakes in combination with a sensible dinner and snacks.

Since Karla had eaten so freely while pregnant, she sometimes struggled to stay on track with her weight-loss plan. But when she felt her determination wavering, one look at her postpartum photos gave her a much-needed mental boost. "I used to eat M&M's almost every afternoon, but I discovered that I could live without them," she says. "That's what those photos did for me."

Ultimately, they helped her lose 41 postpregnancy pounds, leaving her just a pound over her prepregnancy weight 9 months after giving birth. And she's not done yet. "I'd like to get down in the low 130s, and I think I can do it," she says.

As for those postpregnancy photos, they served their purpose well, but Karla doesn't need them anymore. "They're in the closet now," she laughs. "I can't bear to look at them!"

WINNING ACTION

Prominently display your postpartum photo. *If you don't have a photo of yourself from when your baby was born, then get one taken now. Put it in a place where you can see it on a daily basis, perhaps on your refrigerator door,* *your closet door, or your bathroom mirror. It can serve as a powerful motivator in your efforts to slim down. Then as the pounds melt away, get new photos taken and hang them next to the original. You'll have visible proof that your hard work is paying off.*

AT MEALTIMES, SHE LEFT NOTHING TO CHANCE

When Maggie Whitcroft set out to lose the last of her postpregnancy pounds, she wanted to give herself the best possible odds for success. So she created a meal plan to follow every day until she reached her prepregnancy weight. For some, this strategy might seem a bit monotonous. But it gave Maggie the discipline she needed to get rid of her baby fat.

As a mom-to-be, Maggie tried hard to take good care of herself. "Initially, I planned to walk as often as possible, but I ended up not exercising at all," recalls the 39-year-old Scarborough, Ontario, resident. "To compensate, I was very careful about my food choices." She allowed herself just one indulgence: ice cream. "If I hadn't eaten so much of it, I would have done better weight-wise," she says.

In fact, Maggie put on just 26 pounds before giving birth to daughter Nicole in September 1999. That's considered a healthy gain for someone of Maggie's stature—5 feet 3 and 140 pounds. She was down 11 pounds right after delivery, and another 5 a week or so later. But the last 10 seemed determined to stick around.

Home alone with a new baby to care for, Maggie felt that she didn't have the time or the energy to deal with the extra weight. She completely gave up on watching what she ate. "If I could squeeze in lunch, that was considered a bonus," she says. She made dinner after her husband arrived home from work so that he could watch Nicole while she was in the kitchen.

As Nicole got older and established a regular breastfeeding pattern, Maggie realized that she needed to start exercising and eating healthier for herself and her daughter. She added stretches and basic exercises like situps and toe touches to her daily routine. She also created a plan that would take the guesswork out of what to prepare come mealtime. In the process, it would enable her to control her fat and calorie intake, so she could lose the rest of her baby fat.

Even now, Maggie knows her menu by heart. "Basically, I ate the exact same thing every day," she says. "I had a bowl of Special K with low-fat milk for breakfast; tuna with low-fat mayonnaise on whole wheat or multigrain bread and a glass of low-fat milk at lunch; and veggie pasta or a stir-fry for dinner." By sticking with this meal plan, Maggie took off the last 10 pounds of baby fat within 2 months. She has held steady at 140 ever since.

Maggie no longer follows such a rigid meal plan, instead enjoying a variety of foods. But she's careful to control her fat intake and to eat lots of fruits and vegetables.

"I think my strategy worked because I like to feel in control of my life," Maggie says. "Having a meal plan kept my eating habits on course. It provided the structure that I needed to succeed."

WINNING ACTION

Don't leave your meals to chance. *Not everyone could stand to eat the exact same foods every day, as Maggie did. Still, planning your meals for the day, week, or month ahead has definite advantages in terms of weight loss. You have more control of your food choices, so you* *can keep closer tabs on your fat and calorie intake. You're less likely to make a trip to the fast-food drive-thru or to pick up a pizza for a quick-and-easy meal. And if you use your menus to write up your grocery list, you can save yourself time and money in the supermarket— and avoid high-fat, high-calorie impulse purchases.*

THIS MOM FINALLY GOT HER BODY BACK

Two years after giving birth to her daughter, Kate Sarah, Karen Howard still carried most of the 42 pounds she had gained during her pregnancy. She very much wanted to slim down, but like many moms, she just couldn't muster the energy or the motivation to follow through.

Now, 2 years later, Karen is about 26 pounds lighter—just 9 away from her goal weight. For this mom, hiring a personal trainer made all the difference.

Karen wasn't all that concerned about prenatal weight gain when she became pregnant with her daughter. "I just wanted to have a healthy baby," explains the 36-year-old resident of Essex County, England. "I told myself that the weight would come off once the baby was born."

Some of it, about 10 pounds, did disappear rather quickly. But most of it stayed put on Karen's 5-foot-5, 126-pound frame. And the longer it lingered, the more dispirited she became.

"Pregnancy changed my body so much. I was bigger all over!" Karen recalls. "I felt much less attractive. I toyed with the idea of just not eating, so I'd lose the weight quickly. But I knew that wouldn't be healthy for me or Kate, since I was breastfeeding."

Ten weeks after delivering her daughter, Karen went back to work full-time as a lawyer specializing in projects and planning law. With Kate sleeping in 2-hour shifts, Karen had just enough energy to get through the day. In the evenings, she'd crash.

The exhaustion that Karen felt made her even more disgruntled with what she describes as her frumpy appearance. Finally, when her daughter was about 2, she forced herself to go to a gym. "I took step aerobics classes twice a week, but they didn't do much for me," she says. "Being tired really affected my coordination. I could hardly keep up."

Karen knew that she needed help. So on one of her trips to the gym, she asked about personal training. Soon she had her very own personal trainer, who worked with her for an hour twice a week. "Unfortunately, the trainer had no experience with moms who were trying to get rid of their postpregnancy pounds," Karen says. "Her specialty was marathon runners."

Disappointed, Karen went back to working out by herself. Then she met her current trainer, Emma. "She substituted for the instructor in my step aerobics class," Karen recalls. "She seemed really approachable. She even visited me at home. She understood that I needed help, and she was willing to work with me."

Together, Karen and Emma developed an exercise program that would support Karen's weight-loss goals. She did about 20 minutes of aerobic exercise (such as running or cycling), plus strength training for shape and definition. Even though she was working out just twice a week, Karen could see the changes in her body. "My belly was disappearing, and my legs were in better shape than I could have imagined," she says. "For the first time since my daughter was born, I didn't grimace when I looked in the mirror!"

These days, Karen goes to the gym three times a week. She's eating better, too, because the changes in her body have made her more conscientious about her food choices. She figures that she has lost about 16 of her postpregnancy pounds since starting her exercise program. She'd like to lose another 9, which would put her at around 133.

Still, Karen refuses to measure her success by the number on the scale. She just knows that she feels really good about herself. "My stomach is flat, and my legs look fabulous," she says. "Those last few pounds don't matter, because as long as I continue exercising, I can shape my body as I want."

WINNING ACTION

Need help? Hire a personal trainer. *You don't need to be a celebrity to take advantage of the one-on-one coaching provided by personal trainers. Their services are widely available these days. They can help you develop a nutrition-and-exercise plan that matches your unique needs and weight-loss goals. Just as important, they can help you stick with your plan. Virtually all gyms have personal trainers right on staff. Even if you don't belong to a gym, you can call to request a referral. Your doctor may be able to recommend someone as well.*

SHE'S DETERMINED TO DEFY HER FAMILY'S WEIGHTY LEGACY

Adrienne Danke thought the world of her grandmother. After all, they had so much in common. They even looked alike: same eyes, same body type—same weight problem. In her grandma, Adrienne could see herself getting heavier over the years. That was enough to convince her to slim down soon after the birth of her first child.

Adrienne, a 30-year-old Houston resident, has photos of her grandmother in her early twenties. "She was already 'pleasantly plump,'" Adrienne says. "I looked about the same at that age, when I was in college."

Adrienne's grandmother went on to have five children. Each pregnancy left her with a few pounds that she just couldn't lose. Her weight continued to climb as she got older. "She wasn't a very tall woman, but when she passed away in 1989 at age 70, she weighed 275 pounds," recalls Adrienne, who was 19 at the time. "She had high blood pressure in her later years. I could see that happening to me if I didn't do something about it."

Memories of her grandmother's struggle would confront Adrienne years later, when she became pregnant for the first time. "I started out with good intentions," she says. "I struggled with a low-fat, well-balanced diet, since I had nausea 24 hours a day. But I did hold the line on overeating." She gained 35 pounds—appropriate for her 5-foot-10, 147-pound body—before giving birth to son Andrew in June 1999. She lost 22 of those pounds in just 6 weeks, but to her dismay, the rest of the weight didn't budge.

Adrienne thought of her beloved grandmother, who got heavier after each of her pregnancies. "I favor my grandma in so many ways," Adrienne says. "I didn't want to wrestle with my weight all of my life."

Prior to her pregnancy, Adrienne had used diet more than exercise to control her weight. Once she stopped nursing Andrew, she knew that she had to start eating better. She enrolled in Weight Watchers, which taught her the basics of making nutritious food choices and gave her the discipline to eat healthfully. The program helped her lose 13 pounds in 9 weeks.

Today, Adrienne is holding steady at 147 pounds, a weight that she's happy with. "I don't want to be rail thin or model thin," Adrienne says. "I just want to feel good about myself." Her healthy attitude and her commitment to success would undoubtedly make her grandmother proud.

WINNING ACTION

Find inspiration, not consolation, in your family tree. *If a close female relative—your mother, your grandmother, a sibling—couldn't seem to shed her postpregnancy pounds, you may resign yourself to a similar fate. Instead, learn from that person's situation. Talk with her about her experience. Think about what you might do differently to make postpartum weight loss easier, and commit to making the necessary changes. Once you realize that you, not your genes, control your weight-loss destiny, your concern will give way to confidence.*

TRIMMING THE BABY FAT HAS HER FLYING HIGH

The way Bridgett Miller sees it, the men in her United States Air Force squadron did her a favor. By teasing the 27-year-old staff sergeant from Gonzales, Louisiana, about losing her physique once she became a mom, they made her more determined to stay in shape through her pregnancy and to slim down quickly after her baby was born.

In the Air Force, physical fitness is a job requirement. Bridgett worked hard to maintain her 5-foot-7 body at a trim and muscular

129 pounds. Because she was fit from the start of her pregnancy, she believed that she could get back into "fighting trim" soon after her delivery. But some of her colleagues had other ideas. "Two or three guys made comments to the effect of, 'Well, so much for your perfect body,'" she recalls. "They said that once I had my baby, my abdomen wouldn't be tight anymore."

Bridgett interpreted those words as a direct challenge. Intent on proving her fellow airmen wrong, she took steps to control her prenatal weight gain. "I started eating a lot more healthfully," she says. "I gave up fried foods and coffee, and I tried to get more fruits and vegetables, which wasn't always easy. I cut back on dining out, too."

For exercise, Bridgett focused more on low-impact aerobic activities like walking and swimming, which were part of her fitness routine before she became pregnant. She had also been using weight machines, but she cut back on that until after her baby arrived.

If the scale is any indication, Bridgett's efforts paid off handsomely. She gained a healthy 23 pounds before delivering daughter Haley Renee in October 1999, then lost 28 pounds in a little over 2 months. She's holding steady at 124 pounds, slimmer than before her pregnancy.

Needless to say, Bridgett's success stunned her Air Force buddies. "One of them said, 'Wow, you lost that weight quickly,'" she laughs. "I think that's his way of telling me that he was wrong."

WINNING ACTION

Challenge the "conventional wisdom." Like Bridgett, you may know someone who seizes upon every opportunity to convince you that your postpregnancy pounds will become permanent. If you hear those negative words often enough, you just might start believing that *they're true. Instead, use them as motivation to stick with your weight-loss plan and take off the baby fat for good. After all, success is the best—and sweetest—revenge.*

THIS MOM BREAKS FOR BREAKFAST

You can count Gail Place among the growing number of Americans who are discovering the health benefits of a morning meal. Once a confirmed breakfast-skipper, the 30-year-old Pottstown, Pennsylvania, resident began eating in the A.M. because she thought it might help melt away some leftover pounds from her first pregnancy. Now she wonders how she ever got through the day without that all-important morning meal.

Gail admits that she wasn't all that concerned about her weight when she became pregnant with daughter Lindsey, now age 10. "I didn't make any special effort to eat healthfully or to exercise regularly," she says. She would have second thoughts about her attitude after Lindsey's arrival in July 1990. Even though Gail's 35-pound prenatal weight gain was considered healthy for someone her size (5 feet 6, 135 pounds), for her, it felt like too much.

"After my daughter was born, the extra weight just didn't seem to go anywhere," Gail recalls. "So when she was 8 months old, I joined a health club to exercise more. I began to eat better, too."

For Gail, eating better meant adding breakfast to her daily menu. "I was the sort of person who would always skip breakfast, then munch on lots of junk food to make up for it," she explains. "I figured that eating something first thing in the morning would help me do better the rest of the day."

Gail's usual A.M. meal consisted of Cream of Wheat, oatmeal, or low-fat cereal with fruit. She found that as she got into a breakfast routine, her evening meals shrank in size, and she snacked less. "The weight really started coming off!" she says.

In fact, Gail was back to her prepregnancy weight within 6 months. Less than 8 months after that, she lost another 10 pounds.

For Gail, eating breakfast was a total lifestyle change. But it's one that she's glad she made. She has had two more children—daughter Sydney, now 3, and son Zach, who's 1. Each time, she lost the 25 to 30 pounds of baby fat within 8 weeks of delivery.

"I'm convinced that eating breakfast helped me to manage my weight gain through both pregnancies and to slim down afterward," Gail says. Now she can't imagine a better way to start each day.

WINNING ACTION

Put breakfast on your menu. *Research has shown that eating first thing in the morning regulates appetite and discourages bingeing the rest of the day. In this way, it can help you shed those persistent pounds of baby fat.*

Eating an A.M. meal has another advantage: It sets a great example for your kids, who need to fill their tanks, too. Studies have found that children who eat breakfast perform better in the classroom.

You say you don't have the time or the appetite for breakfast? Keep it simple: a bowl of whole-grain cereal, two pieces of whole-grain toast, a container of fat-free yogurt, or a piece of fresh fruit. As long as you get something in your stomach, you'll stoke your body's calorie-burning furnace for the rest of the day.

SHE MADE A SUCCESSFUL RUN AT WEIGHT LOSS

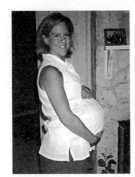

2 days before delivery

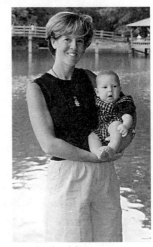

8 weeks after delivery

Kristen Hebert remembers when she thought that people who ran were crazy. "I'd look at them and wonder, 'Why do they punish their bodies like that?'" recalls the 28-year-old resident of Ponte Vedra Beach, Florida.

Now she can answer that question for herself. With some gentle prodding from a friend, she took up running shortly after giving birth to son Chase in July 1999. She had a rather ambitious goal: to compete in a 15-K.

Of course, she also had hoped that training would help trim and tone her postpregnancy figure. She had gained 40 pounds with Chase, an amount consistent with the guidelines of the Bradley birthing classes she had taken. The Bradley program encourages moms-to-be to let their bodies dictate their prenatal weight gain. "It also has the highest rate of unmedicated deliveries, and that appealed to me," Kristen explains.

Still, she worried constantly about putting on too many pounds. "I'd get on the scale backward, so I couldn't see the number," she says. "I'd just ask my doctor, 'Is it okay?'"

It *was* okay, by Bradley standards. Kristen got the reassurance she needed when her 40 pounds of baby fat started melting away shortly after she delivered her son. To help it along, she took power walks on the beach near her home, beginning about 6 weeks postpartum. She also kept close tabs on her food choices. Through 4½ months, she got within 3 pounds of her prepregnancy weight.

Still, Kristen felt flabby and out of shape. She confided her frustration to a friend, who had had a baby at about the same time. The woman suggested that they train for a 15-K together.

Because she had never been a fan of running, Kristen wasn't all that keen on entering a race. But once she started her training, she found that she enjoyed the challenge. And she saw results quickly, even though she ran just two or three times a week in the 3 months leading up to the event.

"My entire training schedule was planned out for me, so I knew exactly what I had to accomplish each day," she adds. "I didn't need to think about it."

Seven months after giving birth to Chase, Kristen found herself standing at the starting line of her first 15-K race, the Gate River Run in Jacksonville, Florida. She surprised herself by averaging 10-minute miles over the course of the race (15 kilometers equals about 9½ miles). "It was an incredible experience," she says. "I felt so good about what I had accomplished."

Now the woman who couldn't imagine why anyone would run is planning for another 15-K, plus a half-marathon. "I enjoy the challenge of training, and of racing," Kristen explains. She also likes maintaining her 5-foot-6 body at a sleek 125 pounds. "I'd like to lose another 5 pounds, but if I don't, I can still look in the mirror and like what I see," she says. "You can hardly tell that I had a baby!"

WINNING ACTION

Challenge yourself to get fit. *If you do the same workout day after day, you just might start to feel like a hamster on one of those little exercise wheels. Such monotony can bring a quick end to your fitness regimen. Add some excitement to your routine by establishing goals for yourself. For example, if you walk at a steady 3½ miles per hour on the treadmill, try working your way up to 4 miles per hour. If you can comfortably do 20 crunches in a row, aim for 25 or even 30. Look for other ways to raise the bar in your workouts. The extra challenge will inspire you to continue exercising—and exercise is key to losing those postpregnancy pounds.*

SHE SHOPPED 'TIL SHE DROPPED HER BABY FAT

Winters in Toronto are cold and snowy, not exactly ideal conditions for launching a fitness-walking program. But Marion Wynter knew she had to do something to slim down after the birth of son Andreas, who's now 9. Otherwise, she feared, her baby fat might become permanent.

Marion had gained 45 pounds through her pregnancy with Andreas. "I was told that I'd lose a lot just from the baby, the fluids, and the afterbirth," she recalls. "But after the delivery, I was just 18 pounds lighter. I was devastated, because I had never carried that much extra weight before."

Determined to slim down quickly, Marion thought that she might start walking with her son. "But Andreas was born in February, so the weather cancelled those plans almost as soon as I made them," she says.

When Andreas was just about a week old, Marion took him along to the mall to pick up some baby supplies. By the time she was done shopping, the weather had taken a turn for the worse. "We had gone to the mall by bus, and I really didn't want to venture outside with him in such nasty conditions," she says. "We ended up staying at the mall all afternoon, walking the upper and lower levels several times over. Andreas was perfectly content to nap in his stroller."

Marion realized that she could do her fitness walking after all, only indoors instead of out. "A couple of days later, we went to another mall and repeated our rounds," she says. "It became a routine for my son and me whenever the weather was bad. On nicer days, we'd do our walking outside."

Within just 1 month of delivering Andreas, Marion lost the last 27 pounds of baby fat. She maintained her 5-foot-9 figure at 150 pounds (give or take a couple) until she became pregnant with daughter Anja, who's now 6. "Unfortunately, I didn't have as much time for mall walking with Anja," she says. "That's probably why I'm still carrying an extra 10 pounds from my second pregnancy."

"I really enjoyed mall walking, for a variety of reasons," Marion, now 34, adds. "I didn't need to buy expensive gym equipment or pay outrageous fees. I didn't need to wait for good weather. I got into shape while spending time with my son. It was good for both of us!"

WINNING ACTION

Do your walking indoors. *The weather outside may be frightful, but that doesn't mean you should cancel your workout. Just head for the nearest mall and do some walking there. The climate-controlled environment is* *ideal for cold- and warm-weather exercise, especially if you have a baby in tow. Some malls open a couple of hours early so that walkers can get in their laps before shoppers arrive. Others sponsor walking clubs. Call your local malls to find out what they have to offer.*

SHE FOUND WEIGHT-LOSS SUCCESS ON THE JOB

The prospect of returning to work after a 3½-month maternity leave weighed heavily on Sylvie Francotte. The 29-year-old Vezin, Belgium, resident treasured every minute with her infant son, Ferdinand. She knew that she'd miss her son terribly, and she worried about not being able to breastfeed while on the job. Over time, she realized that going back to work kept her active and helped her avoid overeating—key factors in slimming down after pregnancy.

Sylvie is employed as a marketing specialist for a company that produces industrial lime in countries around the world, including the United States. She has always loved her job. She is her own boss, and she's constantly on the move. "Keeping busy really doesn't leave me time to think about food and eating," she says. "That has probably helped me to maintain my weight all these years."

At 5-foot-2, Sylvie weighed 141 pounds when she became pregnant with Ferdinand. She gained 18 pounds during her pregnancy. After giving birth to her son in January 1998, she expected the extra weight to quickly melt away. It didn't.

In fact, Sylvie found herself getting a little heavier rather than lighter. She attributed her weight gain to inactivity and increased eating, brought on by just plain boredom. "I was at home with the refrigerator and nothing to do," she says. "So I'd eat something."

By the end of her maternity leave, Sylvie still weighed 147, which was 6 pounds more than before her pregnancy. She found a babysitting service for Ferdinand, and she expressed milk while at work—often in her car or a restroom. That way, she didn't need to stop nursing. "Between nursing and being physically active again, I started to lose weight quickly," Sylvie says. "Getting away from the refrigerator helped, too."

Sylvie became busier than ever, working extra-hard so that she could leave the office on time and head home to her son. After several months, she lost the last of her baby fat, and another 9 pounds for good measure. "I weighed less than on my wedding day," she says.

Since then, Sylvie has had another baby—daughter Josephine, who's just 6 months old. Sylvie took another 3½ months maternity leave, plus a 3-month holiday, to be at home with her little girl. But eventually, she returned to work. It may be her best bet for taking off—and keeping off—the baby fat.

WINNING ACTION

Troubleshoot your move to the mommy track. *When you have a baby, your entire lifestyle changes. That can make losing those postpregnancy pounds more challenging, especially if you're accustomed to an eating schedule or an activity level that's an outcome of your usual daily routine. Be aware of potential "fat traps"— maybe you regularly head for the fridge while your baby is napping, or you spend a lot more time sitting than you used to. Then identify ways to correct such situations.*

Sylvie found that returning to work helped her to slim down. You may think of other options.

FOR THIS MOM, SMALL GOALS LEAD TO BIG SUCCESS

Grace Shickler succeeded in shedding 30 pounds of baby fat. She did it one pair of jeans at a time.

When Grace, a 33-year-old resident of Alpharetta, Georgia, became pregnant in 1995, she didn't worry all that much about weight gain. She knew that the extra pounds would come off eventually. But she also knew that her body would be different. "I had been wearing size 4's, and realistically, I didn't think I'd get in them again," she says. "But I didn't want to keep wearing my maternity clothes either. I wanted a pair of jeans that fit me comfortably."

That gave Grace an idea. After giving birth to her son Jaxson in January 1996, she promptly went out and bought a pair of size-10 jeans. At the time, they were a bit too snug for her 5-foot-4, 122-pound body, which was padded by an extra 35 pounds of baby fat. "I tried them on three or four times a week," she says. "I wanted to slim down to a point where they felt comfortable."

To achieve that goal, Grace continued to eat healthfully—she had always been very conscientious about her food choices—and took baby Jaxson for long walks in his stroller. In about 10 months, she could zip up her size-10 jeans easily. So she set her sights on a new goal: fitting into a pair of size 8's from her college days that, she says, "were broken in just the way I liked."

"I decided to get rid of any clothes that were smaller than an 8," Grace explains. "Pregnancy gave me curves that those tiny sizes would never accommodate." She credits her husband, Scott, with helping her to accept her new, shapelier figure. "He was just so supportive," she says. "He thought I looked great!"

Eventually, Grace was able to wear her size-8 jeans. In the process, she managed to lose 30 of the 35 pounds that she had gained while pregnant. She can still slip into her size 8's with ease.

"Setting small goals for myself gave me something to work toward," she says. "I could see that I was succeeding, and that made me want to achieve more. Now I have a body that I'm happy with."

WINNING ACTION

Establish a series of small goals to advance toward a bigger goal. *If you have a lot of postpregnancy pounds to lose, you need to give yourself time to do it. In that case, your best bet is to take small steps toward your goal weight. Aim to lose 5 pounds rather than 25, or one clothing size rather than four. Once you achieve your first goal, you can set another . . . then another. That way, you constantly feel as though you're accomplishing something. And each small triumph gives you the incentive to raise the bar a little higher.*

CEREAL HABIT SILENCED HER CRAVINGS

Jennifer Rebane has become a cereal junkie. She eats this traditional breakfast food at any time of day, whenever she gets the munchies. She credits her cereal habit with helping her to manage her prenatal cravings and lose 40 postpregnancy pounds.

Jennifer, a 36-year-old first-time mom from Allentown, Pennsylvania, had always taken care to eat healthfully and exercise regularly. At 5 feet 7 and 143 pounds, she was in great shape when she became pregnant in August 1998. Before long, she found herself pining for chips, cookies, and ice cream—foods that had seldom enticed her before.

Jennifer had to eat *something*, but she didn't want to start bingeing on junk food. So she decided to try cereal. "I figured that it would be good for me, since most brands are enriched with vitamins and minerals," she explains. "When you're pregnant or nursing, you need the extra nutrition anyway."

By her own estimate, Jennifer was emptying a box of cereal every 2 days. Her favorites were Total and Quaker Oat Squares, which she enjoyed with or without fat-free milk. "The crunchiness of the cereal appealed to me," she explains. "Besides, it filled me up."

Jennifer also kept up her exercise program, switching from aerobics to walking in her sixth month while continuing with upper- and lower-body strength training. "In fact, I was at the gym one Friday and in the delivery room the following Monday," she recalls.

After baby Sarah's arrival in May 1999, Jennifer began nursing. It made her ravenously hungry. "I had gained 40 pounds during my pregnancy, and I certainly didn't want to gain more," she says. "But because I was nursing, I had to watch what I ate." Once again, cereal saved the day. "It filled me up without a lot of fat," she explains. "And I was getting those all-important vitamins and minerals, which were good for me and for my daughter."

Within 2 months, Jennifer had lost 30 pounds of baby fat, thanks to the calorie-combusting combination of nursing and regular walking—and the craving-crushing power of cereal. At that point, she resumed taking aerobics classes and doing strength training. Six months later, she had taken off another 13 pounds.

Jennifer has maintained her weight at 140 ever since. She no longer gets the cravings that kept her munching during and after her pregnancy. But if she feels the need to snack, she knows that cereal can satisfy her hunger without expanding her waistline.

WINNING ACTION

Make cereal an anytime snack. *If pregnancy or nursing seems to activate your snack tooth, bypass the junk food and pick up a box of low-fat, vitamin- and mineral-enriched cereal. Even the sugary brands help fulfill your body's nutritional needs, making them a great choice if you're dealing with cravings for sweets. (Of course, the healthiest cereals contain the least sugar.) Look for a high-fiber product such as Fruit & Fibre or Frosted Mini-Wheats—the fiber can help prevent constipation. Add fat-free milk for an extra dose of calcium.*

THIS MOM GIVES NEW MEANING TO "HOME GYM"

Aimee Ellingsen never enjoyed conventional exercise. That doesn't mean she's a couch potato—far from it. She prefers to get her daily dose of physical activity by tending to her home and garden. That's all she needed to shed the 24 pounds of baby fat left behind by her first pregnancy.

Aimee lives with her husband, Chuck, and their 18-month-old son, Marcel, in historic New Orleans. Their house is more than 100 years old, with an ever-changing array of repair and beautification projects that keep the Ellingsens busy. "Rather than hiring someone to do the work for us, we do it ourselves," explains Aimee, who's 26. "We're always painting or finishing some odd job."

When she's not fixing up the house, Aimee is likely to be found gardening. She tends numerous rosebushes in her flower beds, plus a large vegetable garden out back. Between them, she has her hands full, pulling weeds and digging holes for planting.

While Aimee was pregnant with Marcel, she did monitor her eating habits and take up walking in an effort to control her weight gain. Once she gave birth to her son, she didn't feel compelled to overhaul her diet or to join a gym to get back in shape. Everything that she needed to slim down was in her own backyard. "When I run on a treadmill, I feel like a hamster in a cage," she says. "If my husband and I want to exercise, we're going to hammer together a lattice or dig a new flower bed. That's how we work out."

Aimee must be on to something, because 9 months after delivering Marcel, she was back to her prepregnancy weight of 114—appropriate for her 5-foot-4 figure. She's not just slim, she's strong and toned, too. "I'm convinced that digging a hole in the garden just might rival crunches," she says. "Afterward, I can feel that my ab muscles have gotten a good workout."

WINNING ACTION

Turn your housework into a workout. *Perhaps you don't have a century-old "fixer-upper," like Aimee. No matter. Even seemingly mundane household chores count toward your daily exercise quotient. And the more vigorously these activities are performed, the more calories they'll burn. For example, the average 150-pound woman can burn 525 calories per hour cleaning the kitchen floor, 345 calories per hour ironing clothes, and*

345 calories per hour washing dishes. That's great news for new moms, who often don't have the time or the energy to go to a gym to work out.

STEPPING OUT SEALED HER WEIGHT-LOSS SUCCESS

Many a new mom is told by well-meaning family and friends to "let nature take its course." Bridget Mann interpreted that advice quite literally. With regular visits to a park near her Minneapolis home, she blazed her own trail to postpartum weight-loss success.

When Bridget became pregnant with her first child, she wasn't all that concerned about accumulating pounds. She didn't make any significant changes in her eating habits or her activity level. "I have five sisters, and for them, pregnancy was business as usual," she explains. "You gain a sufficient amount of weight; you get it off."

By the time she gave birth to son Ethan in August 1999, Bridget had added 27 pounds to her petite 5-foot-1, 103-pound figure. She expected the weight to quickly vanish. But it didn't.

"When I came home from the hospital, I weighed just 5 pounds less than when I went in," Bridget recalls. "It was hugely discouraging. Everyone had been telling me that I'd lose right away. I had never faced a weight issue before."

Since Bridget had delivered Ethan by cesarean section, her doctor advised her to wait 8 weeks before engaging in vigorous exercise. By then, it was autumn, the perfect time of year for walking at nearby Lake Harriet.

The tree-lined lake is one of seven in the Minneapolis park system and a favorite among local residents of all ages. It has its own picnic area, music band shell, and rose garden. But for Bridget, its greatest resource is its walking path. She used it almost every day. After spending several weeks virtually housebound, she welcomed the opportunity to be outside, to soak up the fresh air and sunshine while shedding more of those postpregnancy pounds.

"When you have a baby, getting out is a lot more difficult. You start to feel isolated," Bridget says. "At the lake, I could be around other people and enjoy the outdoors. Walking there became my escape. It saved my sanity."

It also saved her waistline. By December 1999, Bridget had returned to her prepregnancy weight. At age 30, she's expecting her second child, but she's not leaving her figure to chance. She continues to walk Lake Harriet's trails to stay in shape during her pregnancy and to get a head start on slimming down afterward.

WINNING ACTION

Move your workout outdoors. *Whether you exercise outside or in makes no difference in terms of burning calories and melting away body fat. But heading outdoors may have at least one advantage: Many people say that it helps them relax and recharge their batteries. This can be especially valuable for new moms, who can easily feel overwhelmed by caring for a newborn. But any mom can benefit from a little stress relief—and managing stress is crucial to losing weight.*

Virtually every community has a park or recreation area where residents can get in touch with nature. Many have walking trails or bicycle paths, both of which are ideal for low-impact exercise. Contact your local parks and recreation department for more information.

SHE WENT FROM FLABBY TO FIT IN JUST 6 MONTHS

In January 1998, Niamh Dougall could hardly picture herself competing in a triathlon. She had lost fewer than half of the 35 pounds remaining after the birth of her son, Rory, the year before. At 5 feet 2 and 155 pounds, she was well above her prepregnancy weight. She felt out of shape and miserable.

Niamh had taken great care of herself through her pregnancy. But a difficult labor and delivery left her little boy with a disability that devastated her. "I felt overwhelmed by Rory's situation," recalls the 28-year-old Jackson Hole, Wyoming, resident. "My self-esteem fell to an all-time low."

Her sunken spirits bubbled to the surface that fateful January, during a conversation with a friend. "We were discussing how feeling good about yourself can be so hard when you're home alone and you have nothing to distract you from dwelling on your flaws," Niamh says. "My friend mentioned that she had participated in the Danskin Triathlon outside Boston, and that she had gotten a big boost from the experience. She encouraged me to sign up for one."

The event Niamh chose was just 6 months away, in July. At first, she didn't think she could get ready in time. Her usual exercise program—light aerobics and walking her dog—had hardly prepared her for the physical demands of a triathlon. But the more she thought about it, the more she wanted to try. "I had to get in shape anyway," she explains. "I figured that training for a specific event would be better than pursuing a very general goal of fitness."

Once Niamh registered for the event, she knew that she couldn't back out. She bought both a jogging stroller and a baby seat for her mountain bike, so she could include Rory in her training. "Taking my son with me really enhanced my workouts," she says. "I had all that extra weight to push or carry uphill."

Over the course of about 6 weeks, Niamh worked up to running three times a week, swimming twice a week, and cycling twice a week. She became so wrapped up in her training schedule that she scarcely noticed that she was slimming down. Yet by race day, she was a trim and toned 115 pounds. "The weight literally melted away," she marvels. "I couldn't believe how my body changed."

Niamh completed her first triathlon successfully. She enjoyed the experience so much that she trained for and competed in two more events that same year.

Since then, Niamh has given birth to her second son, Aidan, who's now 18 months old. Her pregnancy and delivery went smoothly, and she lost all 40 of her postpregnancy pounds within 6 months of delivery. She has maintained her weight at 115 ever since.

Niamh learned so much through her two pregnancies that she cofounded a Web site, FitMommies.com, to share information with other moms. Even though she's not training for a triathlon, she strives to stay active—and to keep her kids active, too. "I even bought a sled with a cover, so I can tow them behind me when I go cross-country skiing!" she laughs.

WINNING ACTION

Shape up for a specific event. *Once Niamh registered for that triathlon, she had no choice but to slim down and shape up by race day. Perhaps you don't see yourself as a triathlete. No matter. A wedding, a class reunion, or a holiday party can serve as an equally powerful motivator. In effect, it puts you on deadline. You know what you need to achieve by a certain date, and you can measure* *your progress along the way. Just make sure that your goal is reasonable. Aim to lose 20 pounds in a month, and you're likely to end up disappointed.*

SHE'S FIT AFTER 40—
AND FOUR KIDS

Conventional wisdom says that the older you are when you become pregnant, the more difficulty you'll have in reclaiming your prepregnancy figure. If that's true, then Jan Andersen is decidedly unconventional. The freelance writer and humorist from Swindon, England, had her fourth child at age 39—and she dropped back to her prepregnancy weight within 2 months.

Jan had her first three children while still in her twenties. In those days, her featherlight 112-pound figure would return almost instantly. As she got older, she gained 23 pounds—but she remained well within the healthy weight range for someone who is 5 feet 5.

So when she became pregnant with her fourth child, Jan didn't buy into the notion that her still-slim physique would be gone for good. "I wanted to be realistic about it," she says. "But I also wanted to prove that it's possible to have a baby later in life and spring back into shape."

Before her last pregnancy, Jan had been a regular at a gym near her home. But she quit exercising early in her first trimester. "I developed hyperemesis (extreme morning sickness), and I didn't want to do anything that would put additional strain on my body," she explains. The condition also took a toll on her diet. "For the first 5 months, I had trouble keeping anything down," she says. "But I seemed to crave nutritious foods like broccoli, fruit, and fish."

Jan gave birth to her fourth child, Lauren, in November 1999. Over the course of her pregnancy, she had gained 42 pounds. Breastfeeding helped her lose at least some of the weight by burning extra calories. To increase her odds of slimming down, she resumed her fitness routine with the most convenient exercise equipment that she could find: her feet and a stroller.

"I drove the car only when I had to," Jan says. "I walked to friends' homes within a 2-mile radius of ours as well as to the doctor's office and the baby's clinic." When she needed to run errands, she put baby Lauren in the stroller and headed to the nearby shopping centers. And the two of them made a regular pilgrimage to a local park, where Jan did a 3-mile loop before trekking home.

As for her diet, Jan admits that she indulged in her share of chocolate, cake, and other "disgustingly calorific" foods. But she tried to balance them with fruits and vegetables—the foods that she craved during her pregnancy. She also developed a fondness for her daughter's baby food. "I tried not to give in to the temptation to test it or finish it off," she says. "It may look like revolting sludge, but it's actually quite good!"

And it certainly hasn't done any harm to her figure. Two months after giving birth to her daughter, Jan was back to her prepregnancy weight of 135 pounds. She accomplished what conventional wisdom had said she could not do. While she's not as thin as she was in her twenties, that's okay with her. As she explains, "My partner prefers me as I am—voluptuous!"

WINNING ACTION

Prove the naysayers wrong. *Many women believe that once they hit 40, they should just accept defeat in their battle to lose weight. There's no question that slimming* *down and shaping up becomes harder as we age. And bouncing back after pregnancy can be harder still. But that doesn't mean it can't be done, or that you shouldn't try. Just be realistic about it. You likely won't recapture your twenty-something figure, but you can look fabulous with your forty-something curves!*

THIS MOM'S WALLET IS LIGHTER—AND SO IS SHE

Even as her waistline grew, mom-to-be Anne Gentleman found herself tightening her belt. She had to save her pennies for maternity leave, when her employer would pay only 60 percent of her salary.

At the time, Anne was concerned about managing on a smaller income. Now she thinks that it may have been a blessing in disguise. It helped her to eat more healthfully, which in turn enabled her to lose her postpregnancy pounds—and then some.

Anne, a 42-year-old Toronto native, gave birth to daughter Natalia in March 1991. Afterward, she was left with 21 extra pounds on her 5-foot-2, 121-pound body. While she hoped to shed the baby fat, her primary concern was feeding herself and her family healthfully on a smaller food budget. "I had a child to care for and less money to do it," she explains. "That forced me to be more selective in my food choices."

Having a baby in the house also gave Anne less time for meal preparation. She could have spent her money on prepackaged convenience foods—but she didn't. "I preferred to make everything from scratch," she says. "I looked for foods with lots of nutritional value that I could prepare quickly."

On trips to the supermarket, Anne stocked up on inexpensive but healthy items like fruits, vegetables, and cold salads. She bypassed Italian bread, which she loves, in favor of more nutritious whole grain wheat bread. She also bought soups (low in sodium and without additives), juices, and low-fat milk. "I wasn't as concerned about screening for fat and calorie content as I was about getting the most bang for my buck nutritionwise," she says.

All of these foods were easy to prepare, which meant that Anne spent less time in the kitchen and more time with her baby girl. Her smart shopping—and healthy eating—helped her to lose those 21 pounds of baby fat, plus another 16 pounds, in 4 months. She has maintained her weight at 105 since returning to work.

"As my daughter has grown up, I've been careful to set a good example by choosing high-quality, nutritious foods over junk," Anne says. "We feel that we're eating like queens—and we're healthier for it!"

WINNING ACTION

Establish a grocery-shopping budget—and stick with it.
Even though Anne's circumstances were unique, her strategy can work for anyone. Designating a set amount of money for groceries can help guide your food choices, so you buy only what you really need and put back what you don't. Fresh foods tend to be less expensive than prepackaged convenience foods anyway, so you can fill your cart with healthy items and still pay less. Shopping with a grocery list is a good idea, too. It discourages high-fat, high-calorie impulse purchases, the kind that can keep extra pounds around.

SHE WALKS WHILE HER BABY SLEEPS

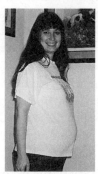

7 months pregnant

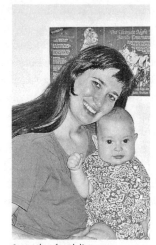

6 months after delivery

The sounds of urban hustle and bustle may not be music to your ears. But they're as sweet as a lullaby to 4-year-old Sylvie Moscovitz. The little girl would invariably fall asleep when her mom, Michele, pushed her in a stroller through the streets of their noisy Manhattan neighborhood. Sylvie got her naps, and Michele got to walk off her postpregnancy pounds.

Michele, who now lives on Long Island, decided to take up walking after Sylvie was born. With a newborn to care for, Michele simply couldn't spare the time to go to the gym—and she had 45 pounds of baby fat to lose. She worried, though, that the constant cacophony of car horns, blaring stereos, and loud voices would make her daughter cry. To her surprise, the little girl slept right through it. "I could push her all over Manhattan, and she wouldn't wake up," Michele marvels.

So while Sylvie snoozed in her stroller, Michele walked—3 days a week, 2 hours at a stretch. Later, as her daughter got older, "I made sure to carry healthy snacks like Cheerios, peeled avocados cut into tiny pieces, and cooked, mashed sweet potatoes," Michele says. "That way, I wasn't tempted to buy junk food en route."

Gradually, Michele's postpregnancy pounds began to disappear. Over the course of a year, she lost a total of 49 pounds. She maintained her 5-foot-3 frame at 112 pounds for 2½ years before becoming pregnant again.

Now awaiting the birth of her second child, Michele, who's 35, is taking a weekly yoga class to keep fit. She plans to resume her walking routine as soon as she's able after her delivery. She only hopes that this baby will be able to fall asleep without the big-city sounds of Manhattan. "Here, on Long Island, it's so quiet that I had to search out a noisier street where I could walk Sylvie for her naps," Michele laughs.

WINNING ACTION

Take a walk while your baby sleeps. *Many experts endorse walking as an ideal postpartum activity. It's gentle and low-impact, yet it burns enough calories to promote weight loss. You can even include your baby in your fitness routine. In fact, if you time your walks properly, you can get your baby to nap while you get your exercise. Just pushing the stroller adds an element of strength-building resistance to your workout.*

SHE REFUSES TO FOLLOW
IN HER MOTHER'S FOOTSTEPS

From age 14, Denise Dewar struggled with a weight problem. Now that she's a mom, she has new resolve to slim down successfully. She knows firsthand the sadness and disappointment that can arise from growing up with an overweight parent. She wants a better experience for her daughter.

When Denise was a child, she missed out on a lot of activities because her mother couldn't take part. "My mom is a very big woman, probably about 350 pounds," explains the 29-year-old Lakewood, Colorado, resident. "She would often say no to things that I wanted to do. I knew it was because of her weight."

As Denise got older, she realized that she might be following in her mother's footsteps. She reached 198 pounds before becoming pregnant, which then added another 16 pounds to her 5-foot-3 frame. "I was very self-conscious about my weight," she recalls. "I hid my body underneath big clothes that draped."

After giving birth to her daughter, Kayleigh, in November 1999, Denise lost 10 of her pregnancy pounds rather quickly. The rest didn't want to budge.

The turning point in Denise's weight-loss battle came the day that she happened to catch a telecast of *The Oprah Winfrey Show*. Oprah's guest was a woman who had lost nearly 200 pounds so that she could do more with her daughter. For Denise, the woman's comments triggered a flood of memories. "I thought about how my mom and I missed out on so much together," she says. "I said to myself, 'I can't do that to my daughter.' I love Kayleigh so much that I never want to say no to her because I'm too big."

Four months after her baby's arrival, Denise had newfound motivation to slim down. To increase her chances of succeeding, she decided to follow the Weight Watchers program. She still winces when she remembers her inaugural at-home weigh-in: 204 pounds.

Weight Watchers taught Denise all about portion control through its POINTS system, which assigns a point value to every food and beverage and a point total to each participant, based on her current weight. So far, she has been able to manage her eating habits pretty well on her own. If she hits a rough spot, she goes online to a moms' group for support. "The women whom I chat with keep me on track," she says.

Besides eating more healthfully, Denise is exercising regularly. She goes for walks with her husband and daughter, and she has taken up inline skating.

In less than 2 months, Denise lost those 6 lingering pounds of baby fat, plus 15 pounds more. She'd like to get down to 135, and for the first time in her life, she believes that she'll succeed. "My daughter is my motivation," she says. "I'm committed to always being here for her."

WINNING ACTION

Defy your family's fat gene. *Research has shown that genetics plays a role in obesity. But it doesn't seal your fate. So don't settle into the mindset that because your family is overweight, you're going to be stuck with post-pregnancy pounds. Someone has to change the pattern; it may as well be you. Besides, by making healthy eating and regular exercise a part of your life, you set a good example for your kids. That may start a new family tradition.*

TO CONTROL HER CRAVINGS, SHE BROUGHT IN THE FOOD POLICE

Aurelia Williams loves salty snack foods. But the 31-year-old Washington, D.C., resident also loves her thin-by-nature figure. So when her cravings seemed to be complicating her weight-loss efforts after her third pregnancy, she knew that she had to stop her out-of-control munching. And she knew just the person to help her do it: her husband, Lance.

The Williamses were thrilled at the news that they were going to become parents for the third time. For Aurelia's part, she saw no reason to worry about her prenatal weight gain. After all, she had already won the baby-fat war twice—with daughter Shayna, now 13, and daughter Isreal, 9. She returned to her prepregnancy weight within 3 months after each delivery. "I never really had to diet," Aurelia says. "I did take the kids for walks, and I think that helped."

By the time she gave birth to son Isaac in December 1999, Aurelia had added 52 pounds to her 5-foot-8, 110-pound body—more than she had gained with her other two children.

She began thinking about the years that had passed between her last pregnancy and this one. "I was older, and my body was slower," she explains. "I realized that the weight might stay on this time." But not if she could help it.

Aurelia scrutinized her lifestyle to see where she might need to make changes to help her recapture her prepregnancy figure. Exercise certainly wasn't a problem, as Aurelia's in-home day-care program kept her in constant motion. Her eating habits, however, were another story.

"I have a real weakness for anything salty—and the saltier, the better!" Aurelia admits. "When things would slow down around here, I'd find myself sitting and munching on snack foods. Especially corn chips, which are the most salty!"

Not knowing how to rein in her cravings, Aurelia asked her husband to intervene. He was more than happy to oblige. "Sometimes Lance would ask me, 'Are you going to eat the whole bag?'" she laughs. "Other times he'd just take the bag away from me!"

Lance's good-natured tactics kept Aurelia's snacking in check. That small adjustment in her eating habits had a big effect: Within 3 months, Aurelia's 52 pounds of baby fat were gone.

WINNING ACTION

Enlist your spouse in your weight-loss efforts. *No adult spends more time with you than your husband. He may be the perfect person to help you shed those postpregnancy pounds—whether by talking you through your unhealthy cravings or nudging you out the door to exercise. Chances are, he will appreciate being asked to pitch in. As a bonus, the two of you might rediscover a sense of connectedness that sometimes gets lost in the hectic weeks and months following a baby's arrival.*

FIBER KEEPS THIS MOM FIT

Scarlett Martin hates diets. The 32-year-old Nashville resident went on one once, and she vowed that she would never put herself through that again. Instead, she found a healthy way to stay slim, a strategy that would provide benefits beyond weight loss, especially during and after her pregnancy.

As a 20-year-old college graduate, Scarlett carried 135 pounds on her 5-foot-3 body. She wasn't exceptionally overweight, but she wanted to be 20 pounds lighter. So she put herself on a very low calorie diet, a decision that she has regretted ever since. "I lost the weight, but it was the most miserable experience of my life," she says. "It made for a very long summer."

Fed up with feeling hungry all the time, Scarlett switched to a new, healthier weight-maintenance strategy as soon as she got rid of those unwanted pounds. She began building her meals and snacks around low-calorie foods that are high in fiber—foods like oatmeal, air-popped popcorn, and black beans. "I learned about the importance of eating healthfully," she says. "I occasionally let my weight creep up 2 to 4 pounds, but never more than that."

By sticking with fiber-rich fare, Scarlett found that she didn't eat as much at meals. What she did eat kept her full for hours, which helped her resist the urge to snack. "Fiber doesn't make me say, 'I hardly ate anything. When's the next meal?'" she explains. "It makes me say, 'That was pretty substantial. I really ate well.'"

When Scarlett became pregnant for the first time, she didn't need to worry about changing her eating habits. Fiber is especially healthful for moms-to-be—not just to control weight gain but also to prevent constipation, a common prenatal complaint. Scarlett put on just 23 pounds while carrying her baby—an appropriate amount for her petite frame. She lost all but 3 of those pounds about 2 months after delivering son Mitchell in August 1999.

Now holding steady at 122, Scarlett has every intention of returning to her prepregnancy weight of 119. She's counting on fiber to help her reach her goal. "It fills me up without filling me out," she says. "I don't need to feel hungry again!"

WINNING ACTION

Take advantage of fiber's slimming effects. *Found in abundance in plant foods—grains, beans, fruits, and vegetables—fiber is among Mother Nature's best weight-loss aids. It makes you feel full, so you're less likely to overeat at meals and to snack in between. And most fiber-rich foods are also low in fat and calories, so they're ideal for anyone who wants to slim down. Fiber has other health benefits, too: It promotes good digestion, lowers cholesterol, and reduces the risk of heart disease. It has so much going for it that you can't afford <u>not</u> to eat it.*

YOU'LL NEVER CATCH HER SITTING DOWN

Baby fat doesn't stand a chance against Kirsi Ratinen. The 34-year-old mother of three from Espoo, Finland, is constantly on the move, switching from one activity to another. Her love of fitness, and her passion for physical challenge, enabled her to get back in shape soon after the birth of each of her children.

During her last pregnancy—with son Pate, who's now 9 (daughter Mari is 11 and older son Timo is 14)—Kirsi ran two or three times a week up until her ninth month. She also took aerobics classes once a week through her sixth month. "We were in the process of building our own house, so I got a lot of exercise just pushing the wheelbarrow and shoveling dirt," she says.

Within 2 months of delivering Pate, Kirsi lost all but 6 of the 33 pounds she had gained during her pregnancy. While on an 8-month maternity leave, she took up Callanetics, a form of low-impact aerobics named after its creator, Callan Pinkney. "I practiced while the baby was napping, or at night while watching TV," she says. "Within a year, I was back to 139, my prepregnancy weight."

While she was very successful in shedding her postpartum pounds, Kirsi needed to redouble her efforts to keep them from coming back. "Once I returned to work, I had very little time to myself," she says. "My family and my job got most of my attention."

Kirsi did manage to go running most days, often while the rest of the family was eating. "I'd make lunch or dinner, then head out the door just as they were sitting down," she says. "I'd have my meal after I returned home." In the mornings, she'd do some exercises from a book called *Yogacise*, by Vimla Lalvani. "Yogacise is a streamlined version of traditional yoga," she explains. "It features a series of poses, or asanas, that can be done in 5 to 10 minutes."

When Pate was 3, Kirsi took up yet another activity: tae kwon do. "I went to class with my son Timo, and I got carried away," she says. "For the next 2 years, I trained the younger kids."

Now that Pate is old enough, Kirsi plans to enroll him in tae kwon do classes. And she'll be joining him. Not that she needs the exercise. "Right now, I'm still doing Yogacise in the mornings, when I'm up for it," she says. "I also do strength training at the gym. And of course, I run." When her schedule permits, she dabbles in aerobics, cross-country skiing, ice-skating, roller-skating, canoeing, and bowling.

Each of these activities provides a unique workout for Kirsi. Together, they create a dynamic and exciting fitness routine that has helped her maintain her fabulous figure—5 feet 6, 139 pounds—since 1992. "I guess I do move around quite a bit," she laughs. "But the variety keeps me interested, which is important. After all, I need to stay active for life."

WINNING ACTION

Let variety add some spice to your exercise program.
Even the most ardent of exercise devotees would find her dedication tested if she had to do the exact same workout day after day . . . after day. The sheer monotony could bring any fitness routine to a quick end. But that's not the only reason to mix and match your physical activities. Look at it this way: If you work the same muscles in the same way all the time, you may unintentionally ignore other body parts that need trimming and toning.

You don't need to be as adventurous as Kirsi to benefit from a varied fitness routine. Try mixing up more basic activities—perhaps walking, cycling, and swimming, or running and strength training.

FOR THIS NEW MOM, A "MATERIAL" GOAL WORKED WONDERS

Most moms-to-be shop for maternity wear. Not Soni Conville. At 7 months and growing, she was buying clothes close to her prepregnancy size. It was all part of her plan for slimming down after her baby was born.

When she became pregnant in August 1998, Soni already had one weight-loss victory under her belt. "I was chubby in high school—I weighed about 127 pounds—and I endured a lot of teasing because of it," recalls the 37-year-old executive assistant from Secaucus, New Jersey. "Then I went away to college, and my schedule kept me so busy that I dropped 25 pounds in about 2 months. I promised myself that I'd never get fat again."

Soni, who's 5 feet 1, maintained her weight at 104 pounds for 18 years. Then she became pregnant for the first time. She admits that she wasn't as vigilant about her prenatal diet as she should have been. "I had severe sugar cravings, and I consistently gave in to them," she says. "I went on a few chocolate binges that are embarrassing to just think about. One morning after breakfast, I ate an entire chocolate Easter bunny, followed by two chocolate cream eggs. That evening for dessert, I had another cream egg, another chocolate bunny, and five chocolate chip cookies—all washed down with a big glass of fat-free milk!"

If her eating habits faltered, Soni made up for it by remaining faithful to her fitness routine. A step aerobics devotee, she switched to walking on a treadmill in her third month, on her doctor's advice. She continued her twice-weekly strength-training sessions, doing exercises for her upper and lower body.

Even though she was working out regularly, Soni worried that her prepregnancy figure was gone for good. "On one hand, I was clinging to the image of a chubby high-schooler," she says. "On the other hand, I was just being vain. I had a closet full of pretty clothes that I wanted to wear again."

That gave Soni an idea. Seven months pregnant, she headed out on a shopping trip and returned home with two beautiful, expensive outfits—both in a 4, just one size larger than she had worn before her pregnancy. "To me, those clothes represented a more tangible goal than a number on the bathroom scale," she says.

Soni was able to continue exercising through her eighth month. By the time daughter Caitlyn arrived in May 1999, she had gained just 35 extra pounds. And she was eager to make them disappear.

With a newborn to care for, Soni had to make some adjustments in her fitness routine. Rather than signing up for a step aerobics class, she went for long walks with Caitlyn in tow. And rather than lifting weights at the gym, she worked her upper-body muscles just by hoisting Caitlyn countless times a day.

As for her diet, Soni did make one noteworthy change. "From indulging my prenatal cravings, I was so burned-out on sweets that I avoided them for months," she says.

Of course, every time she opened her closet, Soni saw those two beautiful outfits that she had bought during her pregnancy. They gave her incentive to stick with her postpregnancy weight-loss program. "With the money I had spent on them, I knew I had to slim down—or else!" she says. They must have done the trick: They fit her, albeit a bit snugly, just 9 weeks after delivery.

Within 5 months, Soni had taken off a total of 31 pounds, enough to get her back into her size 2's. She has maintained her weight at 108 ever since. "The size 4's are big on me now," she says. "But I still wear them occasionally to remind myself that I've reached my goal."

WINNING ACTION

Use your wardrobe as your weight-loss goal. *Many new moms worry about whether they'll ever be able to fit into their prepregnancy clothes. Soni found a great way to turn that trepidation into inspiration. Buy yourself a beautiful outfit and hang it at the front of your closet, where you can see it. Then whenever you feel the urge to indulge a food craving or to skip a workout, head for the closet and take a peek at your new clothes. It just might be enough to keep your weight-loss efforts on track.*

A PHOTO GAVE HER PAUSE

After carrying a baby for 9 months, Kym Jacobs felt that her body deserved a break. She didn't even think about shedding her 34 post-pregnancy pounds for several months after delivering daughter Delaney in August 1998.

"I've seen the photos of celebrity moms leaving the hospital with their babies and wearing their size 4's," says the 28-year-old Lancaster, Ohio, native. "That's just not realistic."

A regular exerciser before and during her pregnancy, Kym went back to the gym when her baby was about 3 months old. She worked out three or four times a week, shaping up so that she could eventually get her instructor's certification in Jazzercise. But almost 2 months passed before the scale even budged.

"I was frustrated, but I tried to stay optimistic," remembers Kym, who at 5 feet 3 weighed 119 pounds before she became pregnant. "For some reason, I couldn't get off that plateau."

With her fitness routine already in full swing, Kym looked for ways to improve her eating habits. She regularly prepared low-fat meals, but she also liked to nibble throughout the day, especially on sweets. "In fact, right after I had Delaney, I went on a major ice cream binge," she admits.

To help curtail her indulgences, Kym dug out a photo of herself showing off her buff prepregnancy body in a bikini. She posted it right on her refrigerator door, so she'd see it every time she went for a snack. "Every time I saw it, it made me stop and think," she says. "Usually, I'd end up saying to myself, 'I really don't need to eat right now.' And I'd just walk away."

Those brief pauses saved Kym from giving in to every craving—and taking in too many extra calories. When she felt genuinely hungry, Kym chose healthier snacks, like low-fat yogurt, fresh fruit, and toast with peanut butter. These minor changes in her eating habits, in combination with her fitness routine, were enough to jump-start her weight-loss efforts. Five months after her pregnancy, the pounds started melting away. Five months later, she was back to 119, where she has stayed ever since.

Now that she's leading Jazzercise classes (she got her instructor's certification in 1999), Kym is even more vigilant about taking care of her body. She still stops and thinks before she snacks, though she does allow herself a small treat every day, such as a couple of Hershey's Kisses or a ginger ale. "It's my reward for being good," she says. "It keeps me on track the rest of the day."

WINNING ACTION

Use visual cues to curb overeating. All of us have been in situations where just the sight of food made us want to eat, even if we weren't hungry. That's the power of visual cues. The right "props" in the right places can actually work to your advantage by reminding you of your weight-loss goals. You can use anything: a photo taken before your pregnancy, an invitation to a wedding, a postcard from your favorite vacation destination. Put it where you're most prone to overeat—maybe in your kitchen or on top of your television or in your office. It will force you to stop and think before you indulge.

THIS MOM MADE
WEIGHT LOSS A CLASS ACT

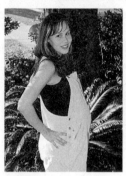

6 months pregnant

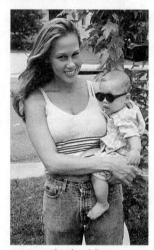

4 to 5 months after delivery

The size-2 jeans seemed to taunt Blaise Harvey. They had fit her 5-foot-6, 115-pound figure perfectly before she became pregnant—before she gained 42 pounds. Would they ever fit her again?

Blaise was determined that they would. And she succeeded, driven in large part by the camaraderie and friendly competition in a roomful of fellow exercisers.

Through her pregnancy, Blaise made every effort to contain her weight gain. She had always been trim, though she realizes now that her eating habits probably weren't all that good. "I used to be psycho about fat-free everything," says the 25-year-old Tallahassee, Florida, resident. "I don't think I ate enough to keep my body at a normal weight."

When she learned that she was pregnant in April 1998, Blaise ditched her fat-free diet and welcomed foods like tuna, peanut butter, and cheese, knowing that the extra protein would support her baby's development. She stopped guzzling diet Coke and snuffed out her cigarette habit. She stayed active, too, enrolling in a pregnancy fitness class and a low-impact step aerobics class. "I thought that working out might help me have an easier delivery, but I went into labor 4 weeks early," she says. "It lasted for 29 hours."

Baby Nickolas eventually made his debut, appropriately enough, on Christmas Eve. And Blaise found herself with an unwanted present: 42 postpregnancy pounds.

Eager to lose the baby fat and regain her prepregnancy physique, Blaise resumed her exercise regimen as soon as she could. "I went to the gym like a maniac," she recalls. Not that she always felt like going. Like any new mom, she had to grapple with the muscle-sapping fatigue that results from round-the-clock newborn care. "But my husband really encouraged me," she says. "Even when I didn't want to go, he'd tell me that I should, that it would make me feel better. And he'd watch the baby while I was gone."

Once at the gym, Blaise drew her motivation from the people in her classes. "I don't like to give up in front of others," she says. "That gave me incentive to keep going, even when I felt tired. Having an instructor to push us and encourage us helped, too."

Blaise continued to eat healthfully, just as she had during her pregnancy. But those regular visits to the gym seemed to give her the edge in her battle against baby fat. One year after Nickolas was born, Blaise was back to her prepregnancy weight—and zipping herself into her size-2 jeans.

WINNING ACTION

Join other exercisers in the quest to purge pounds. *Signing up for an exercise class can provide the motivation you need to start and stick with a fitness program.*

You're bound to meet women just like you, who want to slim down and shape up after giving birth. You can commiserate with each other, encourage each other, and maybe even engage in a little friendly competition. And you'll lose those postpregnancy pounds to boot! These days, even hospitals and churches offer exercise classes. And many gyms offer on-site child care. Check your local newspaper for advertisements.

THE RETURN OF BABY FAT WON'T GET HER OFF TRACK

Ashley Quiamco knows the thrill of postpartum weight-loss victory . . . and the agony of defeat. This 28-year-old mom from Vancouver, British Columbia, shed all of her postpregnancy pounds, only to watch her weight start creeping upward again. Now she's more determined than ever to slim down for good.

Before Ashley became pregnant with daughter Alexey, who's now 3, she maintained her petite 5-foot-1 figure at a trim 105 pounds. She gained 40 pounds through her pregnancy, but the extra weight started coming off almost immediately after delivery. She ended up taking off all of her baby fat, as well as another 10 pounds.

"I remember losing quite a bit when my daughter was about a year old," Ashley says. "Alexey had started walking, and I was constantly chasing after her. Plus, I was under a lot of stress. I'm a single parent, and I work full-time, so my days are very full."

Still, Ashley made every effort to maintain a healthy lifestyle. She chose her foods carefully, building her meals around fruits, vegetables, fish, and chicken. She ran about 6 miles at least 3 days a week, wrapping up each workout with abdominal crunches.

These are the very strategies that many experts recommend for losing weight. They helped Ashley to maintain her slim figure for about a year. Then inexplicably, about 10 pounds found their way back. "I hadn't made any changes in my lifestyle, and I had just undergone a complete physical, which turned up nothing," she says. "I went to my doctor, and she was stumped, too. She switched me to lower-dose birth control pills to see if that would make a difference, since some women get heavier while taking oral contraceptives."

Without a definitive explanation for her weight gain, Ashley couldn't help feeling frustrated. "I wanted to hide," she says. "Even when I tried exercising longer and more frequently, it didn't help."

Despite her disappointment, Ashley has refused to throw in the towel. "My daughter and I lead a very active lifestyle," she says. "We do something active every night, as long as we don't have other plans. We never just sit around, even when we're at home."

By finding ways to keep moving, Ashley has lost 3 of those resurgent postpartum pounds. Just 2 more, and she'll have reached her goal weight of 100 pounds. "That's the weight I feel good at," she says. "I won't give up till I get there."

W I N N I N G   A C T I O N

Never let a setback shake your confidence. *The road to postpartum weight-loss success isn't always a smooth one. After weeks of watching the pounds melt away, you may find them sneaking back. Or you may get stuck at one number on the bathroom scale. Don't let these ups and downs derail your efforts. Instead, remind yourself how far you've come. Ask yourself whether any aspect* *of your life has changed in a way that might stand between you and your weight-loss goals. Use that information to identify strategies that might help stoke your body's fat-burning furnace.*

FITNESS FANATIC LEARNS THAT LESS IS BETTER

Ever since she was a teenager, Lori Vescio has prided herself on staying fit. So when a family member poked fun at her postpregnancy figure, she felt hurt . . . but not for long. She decided to use that unkind comment to her advantage, letting it fuel her postpartum weight-loss efforts. But as she learned, too much of a good thing—even exercise—can be unhealthful.

Before she became pregnant with her daughter Megan, who's now 5, Lori maintained her 5-foot-6 physique at a trim 120 pounds. She had been so active for so long that she couldn't imagine suspending her workout regimen during her pregnancy. Neither could her obstetrician, for that matter.

"I spelled out for him exactly what I was doing—stairclimbing and aerobic weight training for an hour, 6 days a week," recalls Lori, a 31-year-old Des Plaines, Illinois, resident. "He said that as long as I was careful not to get too hot, and as long as I didn't have any pain, I should be fine."

Because of her strenuous prenatal fitness routine, Lori gained just 14 pounds during her pregnancy. Her daughter was a healthy 7½ pounds at birth. While Lori knew that she had to lose some weight—"just enough to get back into my jeans again!" she says—

she felt proud that she had stayed active and fit all the way through her ninth month.

Not long after, at a family gathering, Lori's sense of accomplishment would be put to the test. A male relative, apparently buying into the notion that motherhood ruins a woman's figure, suggested that Lori would never return to her prepregnancy weight. "Basically, he told my husband, 'You can kiss your skinny wife goodbye,'" she recalls. "Everyone within earshot thought it was funny, but I didn't. I had worked too hard to stay in shape."

That unflattering comment rang in Lori's ears for days. It turned her into a woman obsessed, more determined than ever to lose her remaining baby fat. She attacked her workout regimen with newfound fury, adding 15 minutes to each session. "I didn't tell my doctor, because he would *not* have approved," she says. Yet despite her intense efforts, she needed 4 months to slim down to 115 pounds, 5 less than her prepregnancy weight.

In hindsight, Lori thinks she might have been a bit too aggressive in her weight-loss efforts. "I neglected other aspects of my life so that I could work out," she says. "I wasn't eating or sleeping as well as I should have been. I felt exhausted."

Lori had proven herself, and silenced the family skeptics. But she realized that in her zeal to slim down, she could have done serious harm to her body, which was still recovering from childbirth. She remembered that when she became pregnant with her daughter Naomi, now 2. She focused less on losing her postpregnancy pounds and more on spending quality time with her baby.

Even though she cut back on her fitness routine, Lori managed to shed all of her baby fat, returning to her prepregnancy weight of 115. "I really didn't obsess about the extra pounds," she says. "I figured that my body would take care of them eventually."

These days, Lori is back to a full slate of workouts. Her regular schedule includes running on the treadmill, Spinning, step aerobics, kickboxing, Tae-Bo, and light strength training. It seems like a lot, but Lori is extra-careful not to overdo. She wants to stay fit and healthy while her girls are growing up—and for years to come.

WINNING ACTION

Exercise common sense in pursuing your weight-loss goals. *A world-class marathoner takes just over 2¼ hours to cover a 26.2-mile course. Once she has crossed the finish line, she doesn't start planning her next training run. She knows that her body needs several days to rest and recuperate. The same principle applies to you as a new mom. As much as you may want to slim down and shape up, you simply can't go full-tilt on your fitness routine. Your body needs time to recover from childbirth. After all, the duration of your labor probably makes a marathon seem like a stroll around the block! Ease into activity as soon as you can, but don't rush it. You'll have plenty of time for getting fit.*

HER BABY FAT IS GONE, BUT HER CURVES ARE HERE TO STAY

Heather Douglass has yet to reclaim her prepregnancy figure. That's okay with her, because she doesn't want it back.

Not that she wanted to hang on to her 62 pounds of baby fat. She was only too glad to get rid of most of them. But she—and her husband—appreciate the curves that pregnancy left behind.

Heather, a 26-year-old Lakewood, Colorado, resident, was surprised by the number of pounds she gained while carrying her first child. At 5 feet 2 and 123 pounds, she was in great shape when she became pregnant. So she didn't see a need to do anything special to control her weight gain. "I just let nature take its course," she says. "I was pregnant, so why shouldn't I have *some* fun with it?"

Much to her relief, the extra weight didn't hang around long. She gave birth to daughter Payton in January 2000, then dropped to 135 pounds within 6 months.

For Heather, the postpartum weight loss seemed to come naturally, as she adjusted her normal routine to accommodate her little girl. She seldom sat down to a large meal anymore, instead grabbing small snack-size meals when she could. "Payton wanted to be included in everything, so I really couldn't cook or eat unless my husband was at home to watch her," Heather explains. "That alone played a major role in getting me down to my original weight."

As for exercise, Heather hasn't needed to go to a gym to work out. Just chasing her daughter around the house has kept her moving constantly. "Payton requires a lot of attention," Heather says. "She never lets me sit down and rest!"

Even though most of her baby fat has disappeared, Heather's figure has permanently changed. "I realize that my body will never be the same as it was before my pregnancy," she says. "I have hips that I never had before!"

That's not necessarily a bad thing, as Heather has discovered. Her husband, Bryan, and her friends constantly compliment her on her new curves, and that has helped her feel more comfortable with her shapelier figure. "I think she looks great!" Bryan says. "I have a beautiful wife and a beautiful daughter."

Now instead of recapturing her prepregnancy body, Heather's

goal is simply to maintain her weight at 135. With little Payton just entering her toddler years, that shouldn't be a problem!

WINNING ACTION

Acknowledge and accept that your body has changed. *Even if you lose every last ounce of baby fat and return to your prepregnancy weight, your body may never look quite the same as before you became pregnant. You'll notice curves in places that didn't have them before. They're sexy, feminine, and certainly nothing to be ashamed of. Embrace these changes as nature's gift to you for weathering labor and delivery. You'll come to appreciate your slim, strong, sensuous shape—as will your spouse!*

Win the War
Once More

SHE'S A WEIGHT-LOSS WINNER SIX TIMES OVER

With six children ranging in age from 15 years to 8 months, Theresa Thornton has learned to be patient about lots of things. One of them is postpartum weight loss. By letting her body and nature do most of the work, she has slimmed down to her prepregnancy weight again and again.

Theresa wasn't always so laid-back about shedding her baby fat. The 36-year-old Newberg, Oregon, resident remembers joining Weight Watchers 5 months after giving birth to her second child. She was carrying 10 extra pounds on her 5-foot-7 body, and she wanted to get rid of them quickly. She succeeded, but not without making herself miserable.

"Some women love Weight Watchers, but I found it too restrictive," Theresa explains. "In hindsight, I think that I would have slimmed down anyway, even without the program."

That one experience led Theresa to conclude that dieting wasn't for her. She decided that if she became pregnant again, she'd continue her usual routine of eating healthfully and walking occasionally. And once her baby was born, she'd breastfeed, just as she did with her other children. Beyond that, she'd simply let nature take its course. The pounds would come off eventually, she reasoned.

Theresa did get pregnant again—not once, but four times. She consistently gained between 45 and 50 pounds. And all of the weight came off on its own, just as she thought it would.

Theresa concedes that her hands-off approach to weight loss didn't work quickly. Sometimes the pounds lingered for up to 18 months. But Theresa never got frustrated or depressed. "After having so many children, I realized that there's a pattern to gaining and losing," she says. "The pounds do go away. Sometimes they just take a while."

She has no better proof than her own figure. Without fail, she dropped back to 145 pounds, her prepregnancy weight, after her last four children were born. "With my oldest kids, Sarah and Rachel, I wanted the extra pounds gone right away," Theresa says. "With Abbey, Maggie, Elizabeth, and Benjamin, I knew the pounds would go with time. They didn't let me down!"

WINNING ACTION

Let nature do what it can before you intervene. *Once you've had your baby, you can't help wondering when, or if, those postpregnancy pounds will go away. As much as you might want to nudge them along, you don't want to launch a weight-loss program right after delivery. If you're breastfeeding, severely cutting calories can change the nutritional content of your breast milk. And strenuous exercise can be tough on a body that's just been through childbirth. Give yourself time, and let nature do some of the work for you. Come the day of your 6-week postpartum checkup, you may find that most of the pounds have gone on their own. Losing the rest won't seem so daunting after all.*

ANCIENT CHINESE SECRET MADE HER BABY FAT DISAPPEAR

Before she became a mom, Allison Kollmar-Ang had two things that most women can only wish for: the ability to eat anything and never gain an ounce and a mother-in-law who gives good advice. In fact, it was her mother-in-law who tipped her off about a natural weight-loss aid that she credits with helping her to shed 40 pounds of baby fat—and counting!

For Allison, staying slim had never required much effort. "I always loved to eat, but fortunately, I had the benefit of a speedy metabolism," explains the 23-year-old Phoenix-based writer. That didn't seem to change through her first pregnancy, when she added nearly 50 pounds to her 5-foot-7, 142-pound frame. She gave birth to her daughter, Phoenix, in July 1998—and promptly lost most of her baby fat.

In January 1999, just 10 pounds shy of her prepregnancy weight, Allison found out that she was expecting her second child. By the time her son, Trinity, arrived 9 months later, she had regained the 50 pounds—but now they didn't seem so willing to leave. Allison attributed the persistent poundage to a change in her lifestyle. "I went back to work after I had my daughter, so I was always busy," she says. "But after I had my son, I chose to stay home full-time. Sometimes I just ate out of boredom."

As the months passed and the baby fat lingered, Allison became more frustrated and depressed. "I was unhappy with my appearance," she recalls. "I would cry just looking in the mirror. I wanted to wear cute clothes again, without feeling self-conscious."

For the first time in her life, Allison had to fight her own fat war. She knew that winning would require a combination of hard work and willpower. She also counted on a bit of wisdom from her mother-in-law, who advised Allison to drink three to four cups of green tea a day.

"My in-laws are Chinese," Allison explains. "Green tea is an old, old Chinese weight-loss aid. That's one reason why they drink it so often, especially around mealtimes."

Besides adding green tea to her daily regimen, Allison made other healthful changes. She found ways to reduce her fat intake—

giving up meat in favor of tofu and beans, replacing potato chips with pretzels and raw vegetables, and switching from whole to fat-free milk. She started working out, too—albeit reluctantly. "I'm not big on exercising, but I try to do my crunches," she says. "For me, the weight isn't the biggest issue. I'm most concerned about getting things back to where they belong!"

Within 10 months of her son's arrival, Allison had reached 155 pounds, just 10 shy of her goal. "I'll definitely lose the rest of the weight," she predicts. Between her healthier lifestyle and her mother-in-law's herbal weight-loss aid, the odds are in her favor.

W I N N I N G   A C T I O N

Sample the slimming powers of green tea. *Green tea is probably best known for its ability to help lower cholesterol and protect against cancer. But research has shown that it may also support weight loss. In one 4-week study involving 60 obese women between ages 30 and 45, those who took green tea capsules shed three times as many pounds as those who were given a placebo.*

You can buy green tea in tea bag form in health food stores and most supermarkets. If you're sensitive to caffeine, look for a decaffeinated brand. Sip a few cups a day, and it just might enhance your weight-loss efforts.

Note: Green tea may affect a baby's iron metabolism, so it's not appropriate for women who are nursing. And if you're currently pregnant, check with your doctor before using green tea—or any herb or supplement, for that matter.

SHE WORKS OUT
ON "TRIPLET TIME"

After giving birth to triplets in February 1998, Misty Hiatt worried that she wouldn't be able to lose the more than 120 pounds she gained during her pregnancy. To her pleasant surprise, the weight came off rather quickly. Keeping it off was another story.

Misty, a 29-year-old Pensacola, Florida, native, was ecstatic at the news that she was carrying not just one baby, but three. "When you want to have children, and then you find out you're having triplets, that's only more of a blessing," she says. "It's a good thing I didn't know what it took to have one baby when I found out I was having three, or I might have been really scared."

The excitement of pending motherhood soon gave way to concern, as the weight of her growing babies became too much for Misty to carry. Nineteen weeks into her pregnancy, she had to undergo a cerclage, a procedure that closes the cervix to prevent premature delivery. After the operation, Misty had to spend most of her time in bed, for her safety as well as her babies'.

"It was frustrating," Misty admits. "But I was concerned about having babies with lifelong problems from being born prematurely. So the sacrifice was no comparison."

By the time Misty gave birth to Madison, Morgan, and Mackenzie, she had added 123 extra pounds to her 5-foot-3, 128-pound frame. Nursing three newborns helped Misty lose a lot of the weight—about 115 pounds over the course of 8 months. (New mothers burn 500 to 600 calories a day nursing one infant, so Misty was burning about 1,500 calories a day nursing three!) But when she stopped breastfeeding, she had trouble keeping off the pounds. And taking care of three toddlers allowed no time for a regular exercise routine.

"If I tried to go for a walk during the day, something would always come up," Misty explains. "And I wasn't burning enough calories just being around the house, going from room to room, making bottles or washing dishes."

Determined to stop those postpregnancy pounds from creeping back, Misty came up with a way to fit workouts into her schedule. Since the triplets took up most of her time while they were awake, she decided to exercise while they were asleep.

Now Misty wakes up at 5:30 in the morning to go on a brisk, hour-long walk while her grandmother, who lives close by, watches her daughters. Then, after putting her girls to bed at night, she adjourns to her garage to do some work with free weights.

By planning her workouts around her children's sleep schedules, Misty has successfully kept off 115 of the 123 pounds she gained during her pregnancy. While she's maintained her weight at 136 for 1½ years, her goal is to achieve her prepregnancy weight of 128. As her girls grow up and become more active, they'll undoubtedly help Misty stay in shape.

WINNING ACTION

Plan your workouts around your child's sleep schedule.
With a new baby (or three) to care for, you may wonder how you're ever going to find time to exercise. But your child's sleep schedule should allow you to pencil a workout into your daily planner. Ask someone to watch your baby while she snoozes in the morning, then use that time to go for a walk, run, or ride. Reserve your evenings for aerobics or strength training. No matter what activities you choose, you can always free up a few minutes. And even when you're not working out, you need that quiet time for yourself.

THINKING THIN MELTED AWAY 74 POSTPREGNANCY POUNDS

After six pregnancies, Ann Douglas has become something of an expert on the subject. The 37-year-old Peterborough, Ontario, resident even wrote a book about it (called *The Unofficial Guide to Having a Baby*). Like most moms, she has struggled with baby fat—for more than 10 years. So what made her finally start losing? Many things, including, she says, learning to think like a thin person.

Ann is very open about her lifelong struggle with her weight. In fact, she likes to joke that the only time she qualified as *under-weight* was when she was born. With lots of hard work, she did manage to slim down to 142 pounds, appropriate for her 5-foot-6 body. She maintained her weight for 1 month before learning that she was pregnant with her first child.

That was in 1987. Over the next 10 years, Ann became pregnant five more times. And the pounds just kept accumulating. "Unfortunately, I never lost all of the baby fat between pregnancies," she explains.

For the most part, Ann's prenatal weight gain was quite healthy. "During my first pregnancy, I did add 54 pounds, I suspect because I was just coming off a diet and I had an 'excuse' to overeat," she says. Her problems seemed to arise after her babies were born.

To begin with, Ann was just too exhausted to exercise. "Given the choice between hitting the couch and dashing out to the gym during my free time, I must confess that the couch always won!" she says. On top of that, she was extra-hungry from breastfeeding. "I reached for a lot of high-carbohydrate snacks that would give me an instant energy burst," she says. Unfortunately, they also gave her instant pounds.

When her fourth pregnancy ended with a miscarriage in 1994, followed by the stillbirth of a daughter, Laura, in 1996, Ann began overeating to cope with her grief. "I found myself craving chocolate and other high-fat comfort foods," she recalls.

Ann gave birth to her youngest child, son Ian, in September 1997. Sixteen months later, she reached 256 pounds, her highest weight outside of pregnancy. Coincidentally, she was also turning 35. "That milestone forced me to take stock," she says. "I realized that if I didn't start taking better care of myself, I might not be around to watch my babies grow up."

Ann began making all the right kinds of changes in her lifestyle. She used Canada's Food Guide (equivalent to the USDA Food Guide Pyramid) to help her choose healthy foods in sensible portions. She gave up her nighttime snacks and embraced exercise.

But Ann also made an important change in her attitude. "I decided to stop thinking of myself as someone who is doomed to be fat forever," she says. "Instead, I saw myself as a fit person who is temporarily overweight."

With this new perspective, Ann gained new control over her weight-loss efforts. "If I'm having a particularly stressful day, I might be tempted to stuff my face with high-fat foods," she says. "At that moment, I simply take a step back and remind myself that a naturally thin person would find ways of dealing with stress other than diving into a sea of carbohydrates. Then I pretend to be that person."

So far, her strategy seems to be working. In a year and a half, she lost 74 pounds. She hopes to shed 27 more, which would take her to her goal weight of 155. "My kids have told me that they're really proud of what I've accomplished," Ann says. And they should be!

WINNING ACTION

Put yourself in a thin person's shoes. Whether you're staring down a trayful of desserts or contemplating bagging your evening walk, pause to ask yourself, "What *would someone who's thin do in this situation?" You might even imagine posing the question to a particular person, someone whom you consider a role model for healthy living. At the very least, this exercise forces you to pause and think before you make a decision that could conceivably compromise your weight-loss efforts. As a bonus, it may help you cultivate a more positive mindset, which can give you a leg up on weight-loss success.*

PLANNED MEALTIMES KEEP HER SANE—AND SLIM

Maureen McAllister sees her life in two stages: B.T. and A.T. That's *before triplets* and *after triplets*.

B.T., Maureen had a career in the accounting field, with a hectic schedule and erratic eating habits. "I'd have a cup of coffee for breakfast, go out for fast food at lunch, and grab something equally unhealthy for dinner—if I ate at all," explains the 36-year-old Norristown, Pennsylvania, resident.

A.T., Maureen is a stay-at-home mom with a highly structured lifestyle, including set mealtimes. "With triplets, that's the only way to keep my life sane," she says. It has also helped her to lose—and keep off—all 42 of her postpregnancy pounds.

Maureen was already gaining weight when she found out that she was carrying triplets. "My husband and I had been trying to conceive for 5½ to 6 years," she explains. "I took a variety of fertility drugs, which made losing weight difficult."

After giving birth to Shannon, Brendan, and Claire in May 1998, Maureen saw her opportunity to slim down. "I was finally off the medication," she says. "It was the perfect time for me to try to get to the weight that I thought I should be."

As she soon discovered, caring for three newborns would actually help her to adopt a healthier, slimming lifestyle. "Our babies stayed in the hospital for 2 months after they were born," Maureen says. "But once they came home, we settled into a routine."

Central to that routine were regular mealtimes, a big adjustment for a former meal-skipper. "I scheduled three balanced meals a day, plus healthy snacks," Maureen says. "I was eating breakfast, lunch, and dinner, which I hadn't done before I became a mom."

Maureen wasn't just eating regularly; she was also making healthier food choices. "My kids got lots of cereal, fruits, and vegetables," she says. "By feeding them nutritious foods, I was eating better, too."

As for exercise, Maureen certainly got her share. "I'd run up and down the stairs 15 to 20 times a day," she says. "At night, I'd put the kids in their stroller and take them for an hour-long walk. The neighbors loved to see them."

In the 10 weeks after the birth of her children, Maureen's weight dropped from her pregnancy high of 197 to 145—which is 10 pounds *below* her prepregnancy weight. She's been holding steady since 1998, though her goal is to shed another 7 pounds from her 5-foot-7½ frame. She's confident that she'll succeed.

"I tried to slim down before I got pregnant, but I guess I just lost my focus and gave up," she says. "Thanks to my kids, I have a whole new outlook on life. I want to be a healthier mom for them."

WINNING ACTION

Synchronize your family's eating schedule. *Establishing set mealtimes for your family can actually help you slim down. Eating at roughly the same time every day bal-*

ances your blood sugar levels, which curbs cravings and reduces your risk of overeating. It also keeps your metabolism firing at a fairly steady rate.

Of course, as your kids get older, getting everyone to sit down at the table at once can prove a challenge. But if they're taught to adhere to set mealtimes while they're young, they may continue to respect this "family time," even as their schedules become busier.

TO FIND TIME FOR FITNESS, THIS MOM CALLED IN REINFORCEMENTS

Exercise has always been a big part of 36-year-old Jessica Wilson's life. But after she gave birth to twins—one of whom required special care—she had little time or desire to work out. That took a toll, physically as well as emotionally. Jessica's saving grace was hiring a helper for a few hours a week. It freed her to go to the gym, where she found stress relief, solace—and a slim waistline.

At 5 feet 6 and 120 pounds, Jessica was in excellent shape before she became pregnant. Living in Japan at the time, she walked every day (she didn't have a car) and performed a type of Japanese drumming called taiko for 2 hours, three times a week. "It's a very physically demanding sport, as well as an art," she explains. "It helped me stay trim and toned."

Through her pregnancy, Jessica continued walking regularly. She also practiced prenatal yoga until a week and a half before giving birth. She gained a total of 65 pounds—most of it baby and water weight. "Even though people said that I didn't look like I was

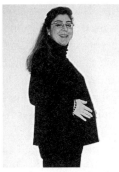

4 months pregnant with twins

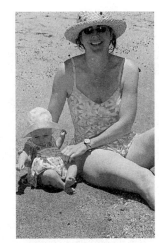

4 months after delivery

carrying twins, I felt huge," she says. "I couldn't climb the stairs without losing my breath. My thighs were rubbing together."

Jessica delivered Rebecca and Noah by cesarean section on March 1, 1999, which was 7½ weeks before their due date. Both babies had to stay in the hospital: Rebecca for 25 days, and Noah, who was born with a hole in his diaphragm and compromised lung function, for 60 days.

"My husband and I were under a lot of stress," Jessica recalls. "We were constantly driving back and forth to the hospital, and we didn't know if Noah would survive. I would sneak peanut M&Ms and malted milk balls into the hospital to munch at my babies' bedsides. Eating helped me to deal with the stress."

Unfortunately, it also helped to widen her waistline. Over the course of a month or two, Jessica regained 20 of the 60 pounds that she had lost right after delivery.

To add to her stress, she and her husband relocated to Elk Grove, California, when the twins were just 5 months old. In her new hometown, she had no family or friends to lean on. And little Noah still needed special care. He was hooked up to a feeding tube, and he had to be rushed to the emergency room several times.

Jessica became so distraught about her situation that she finally went to her doctor. "I was crying constantly, and I couldn't bear to continue on that way," she recalls. "I realized that if I didn't start going to a gym again, I would lose my mind. Exercising is the one thing that gives me a sense of control."

Before she could resume her workouts, Jessica had to find someone to watch the twins. With no family or friends in the area, she decided to hire a nanny.

For 2 hours each weekday morning, Jessica has been leaving her kids in their nanny's care and heading for the gym. The brief reprieve has given her a chance to work off her stress and lift her spirits. "Going to the gym changed my world," she says. "My depression subsided, and my energy level kicked up. I got stronger, and I slept better. My whole attitude changed."

So did her figure. With regular exercise, Jessica dropped to a fit and muscular 138 pounds in just 6 months. She has held steady ever since—and she looks and feels better than ever!

WINNING ACTION

Ask for help with the kids, so you can take time for yourself. *Many new moms would rather forgo their fitness routines than spend even a half-hour away from their children. You need that time, and not just to support your weight-loss efforts. Working out does wonders for your mental and emotional health, relieving stress and boosting your mood. You'll feel more energized and upbeat when you return home.*

If your spouse isn't able to watch the kids, you may want to hire a nanny, as Jessica did. Or consider swapping babysitting duty with a friend or neighbor who has young children.

SHE WROTE THE BOOK ON WEIGHT-LOSS SUCCESS

Lisa E. Davis gained more than 40 pounds during each of her two pregnancies. Both times she managed to shed her baby fat—and then some—simply by putting pen to paper.

Even as a child, Lisa had healthy eating habits. They helped keep her trim all the way through high school. Once in college, she gained 10 of the notorious "freshman 15." But she lost those pounds within 3 months of graduation by adding a 30-minute jog to her daily routine.

In fact, Lisa felt she was in fantastic shape—5 feet 5 and 148 pounds—when she became pregnant with her first child. But over the course of her pregnancy, she gained 42 pounds, putting her close to the 200 mark by the time she delivered. "For the first time in my life, I felt fat," recalls the 41-year-old attorney from South Orange, New Jersey.

In December 1997, about 5 months after giving birth to her son, Marcus, by cesarean section, Lisa decided that she needed a little help with her postpregnancy weight loss. So she enrolled in Weight Watchers for Nursing Women. The program's weekly weigh-ins kept her motivated, and its emphasis on portion control kept her calorie intake down. But what helped Lisa most in her pursuit of weight-loss success was learning to keep a journal.

After each meal, Lisa would jot down what she had consumed, paying special attention to details like how many servings she had eaten from each food group and how much water she had drunk. She also documented each of her exercise sessions, noting whether her workout was the strength-building kind or the huff-and-puff aerobic kind.

"Writing everything down really kept me on track," Lisa says. "I was able to compare my journal from week to week and quickly identify where I needed to make adjustments in my eating habits or exercise routine. If I lost 3 pounds one week and gained ½ pound the next, I could refer to my journal to learn what I was doing right—and what I was doing wrong."

Guided by her journal, Lisa lost 50 pounds within 10 months, dropping below her prepregnancy weight. When she became pregnant again, however, she gained all those pounds back, and then some. But this time, she knew what to do to get rid of them.

Shortly after giving birth to daughter Noëlle in January 2000, Lisa rejoined Weight Watchers for Nursing Women. And of course, she kept her eating-and-exercise journal. Within 7 months, she lost 51 pounds, leaving her just 10 pounds shy of her goal weight of 135.

For Lisa, the rewards of losing her baby fat have gone beyond reclaiming her prepregnancy physique. She feels more energetic, and she looks years younger. "Who wants to look like a 40-year-old woman with two kids?" she muses. "I'd rather look like a woman in her early thirties who *might* be a mom—though you can't be sure!"

WINNING ACTION

Keep a written record of your eating and exercise habits.
The next time you're in a bookstore or greeting card shop, spend a few dollars on one of those pretty journals. Then

use it to track your eating habits—what you eat or drink and when, as well as how you feel at the time (stressed or blue, for example). Also note any physical activity that you engage in. By writing down all of this information, you can identify behaviors that may be impeding your weight-loss efforts. Just as important, you can see what you're doing right—and reward yourself for it.

HEALTHY BABIES MEAN MORE TO HER THAN BABY FAT

Rose Rogari works as a product manager in the information services division of a major telecommunications provider. Even though she faces constant pressure on the job, she has learned to deal with it. Perhaps that's because it pales in comparison with the persistent stress and anxiety of going through two high-risk pregnancies.

At 5 feet 7 and 125 pounds, Rose seemed the picture of health. She never expected to have trouble conceiving or carrying her children to term. So when her first two pregnancies ended in miscarriage, she and her doctor knew that something was wrong. "I found out that I had a uterine anomaly and a progesterone deficiency, both of which contributed to my two miscarriages," says the 40-year-old Archbald, Pennsylvania, resident. "My doctor told me that if I got pregnant again, I'd have to keep my activity to a minimum."

Rose did get pregnant again—not once, but twice. Following her doctor's orders, she all but stopped exercising. And she watched as her weight ballooned. In fact, she gained 60 pounds with both of her daughters (Mia, now age 9, and Gianna, age 7). That's well above the 28 to 40 pounds recommended for someone her size. "My doctor told me that I was okay as long as I didn't develop high blood pressure or gestational diabetes," she notes.

Through both of her pregnancies, Rose's top priority was to keep her babies healthy. But she promised herself that she'd resume exercising just as soon as she could after her babies were born. She kept her word, enrolling in a step aerobics class within weeks of each daughter's arrival.

"I went faithfully three times a week for the full 3 months of the class," Rose says proudly. "It really helped me to regain my prepregnancy figure. I lost all of the extra pounds within 3 months of delivering Mia and within 2 months of delivering Gianna."

In fact, Rose had extra incentive to slim down after Gianna was born. Rose's brother was getting married just 3 months later, and she was a bridesmaid. "I wanted to be sure that I looked as good as everyone else," she says. "On days when I didn't feel like exercising, that kept my motivation strong."

Along with her step aerobics classes, Rose made a significant dietary change, switching to vegetarianism after Gianna was born. "Because I'm no longer eating meat, I make sure to get enough protein in my diet," she says. "I eat peanut butter, as well as low-fat yogurt, cheese, and nuts. My daughters aren't vegetarian, but they like their veggie burgers, too."

Rose credits her combination of a vegetarian diet and regular exercise with helping her to regain and maintain her prepregnancy figure. She has held steady at 125 pounds for more than 7 years. "Giving up exercise during my two pregnancies was tough, but I'd do it all over again," she says. "My daughters were worth it!" To be sure, her pregnancies had their challenges. But they've made motherhood all the more special.

W I N N I N G   A C T I O N

Ease back into exercise as soon as you're able. *As Rose learned, the rules of pregnancy change once you're identified as high-risk. Physical activity is often limited, if not banned completely. And that can lead to greater-than-expected prenatal weight gain. Rather than worrying about your waistline, focus on keeping your baby healthy and make plans to resume your workouts after delivery. Most doctors recommend a 6-week window between giving birth and getting back into a regular exercise routine. In the meantime, keep reminding yourself that the baby fat won't be around forever. If you follow your doctor's advice during and after pregnancy, the pounds* <u>will</u> *come off.*

AFTER SIX KIDS, SHE'S SLIMMER THAN EVER

If any mom could make a case for not having time to exercise, it's Terie Wiederhold. The 36-year-old Provo, Utah, resident has six children ranging in age from 3 to 16, plus two foster kids. She's on the go virtually every waking minute. Still, she manages to squeeze in a workout 5 days a week. Not only that, she actually weighs 10 pounds less than she did before starting a family.

How does this ultra-busy mom fit exercise into her daily routine? Simple: She works out at the same time on designated mornings, just as though it were a standing appointment on her schedule.

To guard against interruptions, Terie rolls out of bed at 5:30

A.M., long before the rest of her family. "I get up no matter how tired or worn out I feel," she explains. "I have to, or I won't work out. I'll be too busy with the kids, or I'll just forget."

Terie has followed this routine for about 10 years, ever since her third pregnancy. "I used to take step aerobics classes, but now I run," she says. "I put in 2 to 4 miles a day, 5 days a week." She eases up on her routine when she's pregnant, but she doesn't stop exercising altogether. "In fact, with my last three kids, I worked out right up until the day of delivery," she says. "Then 2 to 3 weeks later, I was back at it."

Over the course of six pregnancies, Terie has gained a total of 160 pounds—and lost 170. "I usually need about a year to shed all of the weight," she says. "But the older I get, and the more kids I have, the longer it takes to slim down."

After giving birth to her youngest child, daughter Serena, in January 1998, Terie dropped down to 145 pounds—a healthy weight for her 5-foot-7 frame, and 10 pounds less than before she started her family. "I exercise regularly, and I try to watch what I eat, though that's not always easy, because I love food," she says.

Serena and her siblings—16-year-old Curtis, 14-year-old Crystal, 11-year-old Micah, 8-year-old Marissa, and 4-year-old Brea, plus 19-year-old Ethan and 4-year-old Mikayla—can be proud of their mom. She's more fit now than she has ever been. "My goal is just to stay in shape," she says. "As long as I'm sticking with my schedule and exercising regularly, I feel good about myself."

WINNING ACTION

Schedule your workouts on your calendar. If you're serious about shedding those postpregnancy pounds, you absolutely must find time for exercise. Many experts rec-

ommend blocking out 30 minutes to an hour of each day expressly for that purpose. Write it in your calendar, then treat it just as you would an appointment with your doctor or your boss. Gradually, your workouts will become an integral part of your daily routine. You won't even need to ask yourself, "Do I really want to exercise today?" You'll just do it. You'll come to respect that time as your own—and so will your family.

FAMILY KEEPS HER FOCUSED ON FITNESS

Coneen Brace firmly believes that "mother knows best." That's why she turned to her mom for advice when she had to lose some post-pregnancy pounds—not once, but four times.

Through each of her four pregnancies, Coneen added between 20 and 29 pounds to her 5-foot-8½, 160-pound frame. She says that she never made any significant dietary changes while expecting. "I tried to be careful about my food choices, but that wasn't always easy, because moms so often eat on the run," explains the 37-year-old Hutto, Texas, resident. "If I craved a particular food, I ate it. But I stopped when I was no longer hungry."

As for exercise, Coneen didn't see the need for a formal fitness program either. "With five kids between ages 2 and 13 (the oldest, Alexandra, is her stepdaughter), I'm constantly on the go," she says.

Even though she didn't do anything special to manage her prenatal weight gain, Coneen lost most of her baby fat fairly soon after each delivery. Like many moms, she usually had a few persistent pounds to contend with. But she believed that her mother would know how to get rid of them. She was right.

"My mom is a huge factor in my life," Coneen explains. "She inspires me to be a better wife, mother, and sister." She also knows what it's like to need to slim down. "Mom was a little chubby after having her kids," Coneen says. "But with good nutrition and exercise, she took the weight off and has kept it off all these years."

When Coneen wanted to lose her baby fat, her mother gave her the motivation to succeed. "Every time we'd talk about my changing my eating habits or establishing a regular fitness program, I'd say something like 'I'll start on Monday,'" Coneen recalls. "And she'd say, 'Then you just don't want to do it badly enough!' That really spurred me on."

Coneen's husband, Wesley, also served as a morale booster in her battle against baby fat. "He's a lieutenant in our local fire department, so he has to stay in great shape," Coneen explains. "He works at it—he's very active. If he weren't taking such good care of himself, it would be a lot easier for me to binge on a carton of ice cream."

Since the Braces would like to add to their brood, Coneen expects to be fighting a few more baby-fat wars to maintain her weight at about 160 pounds. With her mom and husband to motivate her and cheer her on, she's confident that she'll be victorious.

WINNING ACTION

Find a role model in your family tree. *You likely have at least one relative—mother, sister, even an aunt or a cousin—who has managed to slim down successfully after pregnancy. Ask her how she did it. She'll be able to offer unique insights into issues like dealing with prenatal* *cravings or fitting in exercise after the baby is born. She might even be willing to become your personal coach, keeping you on track for success.*

THE THIRD TIME WAS THIS MOM'S WEIGHT-LOSS CHARM

During times of stress, Sue Upmann invariably turned to food for comfort. It lifted her spirits, but it also filled out her figure. So when the Stoughton, Massachusetts, resident became pregnant with her third child, she seized upon the opportunity to take control of her eating habits and her weight gain. She did both with such success that she now weighs less than she did before starting a family.

At her heaviest, Sue carried 235 pounds on her 5-foot-3 frame. Some of those pounds were leftovers from her pregnancies with sons Tyler, now age 5, and Dillon, age 3. But she knew that she couldn't pin her problem solely on prenatal weight gain, since she didn't put on that many pounds while pregnant. She believed that stress eating bore most of the blame.

"Any stressful event—a bad day with the kids, a spat with my husband—could make me overeat," she recalls. "I wouldn't even stop to think about what I was putting in my mouth."

When Sue found out that she was expecting her third child, the prospect of putting on even a few more pounds gave her pause. "I was tired of being overweight," she says. "I was tired of being tired."

Sue vowed to make this pregnancy different. She would take steps to minimize her prenatal weight gain, so she wouldn't end up with a lot of extra pounds afterward.

Sue's first task was to change her diet. Her midwife advised her to eat more lean protein and to cut back on fat wherever possible. "She also told me to drink water like I was never going to get another drop," Sue laughs. "It kept me in the bathroom, but it also made me more awake and energized. I felt like I was flushing the fat from my body."

As for exercise, she tried to walk as much as she could. "But even when I couldn't get out, just chasing after my boys kept me active," she says.

Sue's strategies worked—perhaps a bit too well. She gained only 4 pounds through her pregnancy, well below the recommended 15 for a woman her size. But her midwife wasn't concerned, since the baby was developing normally and Sue was eating well-balanced meals.

After giving birth to son Jared in May 1999, Sue quickly lost her prenatal weight plus a few extra pounds, dropping to 225. But she wanted to go even lower. A year later, she got the opportunity through her local chapter of the MOMS (Moms Offering Moms Support) Club, an international support group for stay-at-home mothers. "One of our members is also a Weight Watchers leader, and she set up a program for those of us who were interested in shedding some pounds," Sue explains. "I jumped at the chance. Combining the two activities—the MOMS Club and Weight Watchers—was so convenient."

Weight Watchers taught Sue the basics of good nutrition, so she could make healthier food choices. "I'm getting much more fiber than I used to," she says. "I love beans, so I'm eating lots of those. And I'm always snacking on baby carrots and cucumbers." She made changes in her cooking, too. "My husband and my two older sons loved Hamburger Helper," she says. "Now they're getting more chicken, and they love it just as much."

Just one obstacle remained between Sue and a healthy diet: her tendency to binge during times of stress. She knew that she couldn't stop her cravings completely. But she could pay more attention to what she was eating and, more important, *why*. "Now when I feel stressed and I get the urge to eat, I tune in to my body," she says. "I drink a big glass of cold water to see if that stops my craving. If it doesn't, I think about what I'm hungry for and try to come up with a healthy compromise. If I want chips, I'll eat pretzels instead. If I want ice cream, I'll eat yogurt."

Sue's think-before-you-eat technique, along with her other re-vamped eating habits, has taken her down to 208 pounds. And she isn't done losing yet. Now expecting her fourth child, she has every intention of eating healthfully while pregnant. And once she has had her baby, she'll resume working toward her goal weight of 140 pounds.

"As much as I want the weight to be gone, I understand that I need to be patient," says Sue, now age 35. "I tell myself that next month, next year, I'll weigh less than I do right now. That keeps me focused."

WINNING ACTION

Think twice about why you're eating. *Some experts like to distinguish between hunger and appetite—the former being a physical need for nourishment, the latter resulting from some emotional trigger. Stress, anger, depression, and boredom can easily bring on a binge. These emotions are common among moms, who may feel as though they're being pulled in a thousand different directions. When you have the urge to eat, stop and think about what's driving your desire. Are you genuinely hungry? Or are you experiencing some sort of emotional upset?*

Follow Sue's lead and drink a glass of water to see if it quiets your craving. If it doesn't, at least you're making a conscious decision about whether and what to eat. That awareness may be enough to rein in your binge.

SHE OUTRAN STRESS—AND HER POSTPREGNANCY POUNDS

With three children under the age of 6, Monica Hingst faces her share of daily stresses. But she knows just what to do for relief: She laces up her running shoes.

While Monica took up running relatively recently, fitness is nothing new to the 34-year-old Memphis resident. She became an aerobics instructor while a senior in college, and over the years, she has taught everything from high-impact aerobics to step aerobics to kickboxing. And she has no intention of stopping.

Once she began having children, Monica decided to add running to her exercise program. She even had a specific goal in mind: to compete in a marathon. She started out by entering a 16-mile race just 7 months after giving birth to daughter Abigail in February 1997. Two years and another baby—daughter Emma—later, she ran in a half-marathon. She did her first full marathon in December 1999, and another in October 2000.

For Monica, these races provided extra motivation to stick with her exercise program. Even though she had been working out regularly for years, motherhood made it more of a challenge. "Sometimes I felt so tired that I didn't want to run," she says. "And I very well may not have if I hadn't been in training for a race. That's what kept me going."

At first, Monica ran solely to stay in peak physical condition. But the more miles she logged, the more she valued another of exercise's many benefits: stress relief. "My workout is my time alone," she says. "For an hour or so, I don't need to worry about dirty diapers and spilled apple juice. I've come to treasure that. It has provided some peace and serenity."

Between running 5 days a week and teaching aerobics classes, Monica hasn't allowed the baby fat to settle in on her trim 5-foot-4 physique. She gained 26 pounds through each of her three pregnancies and lost all of the weight within 3 months of delivery. Now at 130, she weighs just 6 pounds more than she did before having son Matthew in July 1995.

Monica certainly appreciates what exercise has done for her body, but she also values what it does for her mind. "When the kids are having a bad day and the house is in a wreck, I can't wait to go out running," she says. "And once I'm done, I feel better—like I can deal with anything." That's a feeling that any mom would welcome!

WINNING ACTION

Soothe your spirits while slimming your waistline. *When you're under stress, you may feel too tired or pressed for time to exercise. That's precisely when you should slip into your sweats and work out. Physical activity triggers the release of feel-good brain chemicals called endorphins while burning off stress chemicals such as adrenaline. In other words, it lifts your mood and relaxes your body while melting away those postpregnancy pounds. As a bonus, it wards off stress-induced eating, a common cause of weight gain.*

SHE TRADED IN
HER SIZE 28'S FOR 12'S

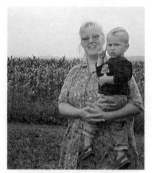

1 year after delivery of second child

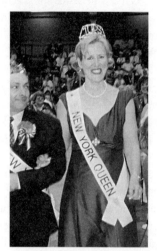

1 year after delivery of third child

Plenty of women would jump at the chance to buy themselves a brand-new postpregnancy wardrobe. Not Laurie Slawta. Her prepregnancy clothes suit her just fine. "It's them or my maternity clothes—or nothing at all," she says. "And the latter two options would be excruciatingly embarrassing!"

For Laurie, a 36-year-old stay-at-home mom from Newark Valley, New York, her prepregnancy wardrobe—stocked with size 10's and 12's—is an ever-present reminder of her past weight-loss success. It also served as a powerful motivator to shed the 25 pounds left behind by her third pregnancy.

After the births of her first two children—Levi, who's now 8, and Ben, who's 6—Laurie was left carrying 289 pounds on her 5-foot-9 frame. "I hurt all over," she recalls. "While I probably could have lived with that, I couldn't have lived with my children's disappointment when I told them that I wasn't able to run, tumble, and play with them."

With a family history of both adult-onset (type 2) diabetes and breast cancer, Laurie had another good reason to slim down. "I knew that obesity is a risk factor for both of these diseases," she says. "I realized that I had to take control of my weight."

Laurie joined TOPS (Take Off Pounds Sensibly), which taught her to make healthy food choices and encouraged her to exercise regularly. Within 2 years, she managed to lose 120 pounds. She maintained her weight for 1½ years before becoming pregnant for a third time.

After giving birth to daughter Claire in June 1999, Laurie was 25 pounds above her prepregnancy weight—and determined to shed every extra ounce. "I lost 17 pounds within the first week, but the last 8 hung around for 8 more months," she says. "I was breast-feeding, and Claire was gaining weight slowly. So my doctor advised me to add a bit more fat to my diet."

During those 8 months, Laurie never lost sight of her weight-loss goal. In fact, she didn't need to look any further than her closet. "I had already given away all of my size 28's, and I was left with only 10's and 12's," she explains. "I realized that if I bought new clothes in a larger size, they'd only camouflage the fact that I was over my ideal weight. And they'd give me extra room, so more pounds could creep on. I made up my mind not to buy any new clothes until I could wear my old ones again!"

Laurie has been back in her size 12's since February 2000. She credits the advice and support she received through the TOPS program with helping her to reach her prepregnancy weight of 169 pounds—and her wardrobe with helping her to maintain her weight-loss success.

She also credits motherhood with giving her a healthier perspective on life. "So much of what I thought mattered really doesn't, in the grand scheme of things," she says. "I have a lifetime to do dishes, but only a few precious years to tuck my kids into bed at night. Motherhood has taught me what's really important, and what's just lint!"

WINNING ACTION

Open your closet for weight-loss inspiration. *The fit of your prepregnancy clothes can be a more accurate measure of your weight-loss success than the number on your bathroom scale. It can also be a powerful motivator, keeping you focused on your weight-loss goal. Perhaps you have a favorite outfit that you want to wear again. Hang it at the front of your closet, where you'll see it often.*

MODERATION WORKED MAGIC ON HER WAISTLINE

As a competitive swimmer and triathlete, Maria Fisher always believed that her super-active lifestyle had helped her to slim down after her first two pregnancies. Then a family crisis forced her to suspend her athletic training 6 months into her third pregnancy. But she still managed to curb her prenatal weight gain, an achievement that she credits to her anything-in-moderation attitude toward food.

Maria, a 35-year-old Farmington, Utah, native, has always been a fitness buff. So when she and her husband decided to start a family, she never considered giving up her training schedule. With her doctor's approval, she planned to continue working out through the third trimester of each pregnancy. She kept to her promise, swimming five times a week while carrying daughter Heather (now age 8), and swimming and strength training five times a week with son Connor (age 6).

Through both pregnancies, Maria added no more than 30 pounds to her 5-foot-5 body. And she was back to 120, her prepregnancy weight, within 6 months of each delivery—an achievement that she attributed to the calorie-burning combination of exercise and breastfeeding.

When Maria became pregnant with her third child, she changed her fitness formula slightly, taking aerobics classes instead of swimming and continuing weight training. All seemed to be going well until her sixth month, when she and her husband received the devastating news that Connor had Ewing's sarcoma, a highly malignant form of cancer. "I gave up exercising altogether, so I could concentrate on his treatments," she recalls.

Shortly after daughter Amber arrived in January 1997, Maria and her husband took turns staying at the hospital with Connor, who was undergoing a bone marrow transplant. "We practically lived there," she says. "Between caring for a newborn and spending my days with our son, I was quite exhausted mentally and physically. I didn't have much energy for anything else, including exercise."

Maria did squeeze in 20 minutes on a treadmill once or twice a week—"but that was only to relieve the stress of my son's illness," she explains. "I wasn't even thinking about getting back in shape." So she was quite surprised when she lost her 30 postpregnancy pounds, just as she had done before—only this time, without the benefit of a workout regimen.

How did she do it? Maria credits her eating habits, which have remained constant during and after all of her pregnancies. "While I'm careful about my fat intake, I don't believe in depriving myself of anything," she says. "In the summer, I love to eat fresh fruit. But I also enjoy snacking on ice cream, popcorn, and cookies with the kids."

Maria is convinced that by allowing herself sensible portions of whatever foods she wants, she avoids the intense cravings that can lead to overeating and weight gain. "I've never believed in dieting," she says. "My motto is 'Anything in moderation.'"

As for her workout regimen, Maria didn't even consider resuming her training until 1½ years after her son's diagnosis. "It wasn't that I wanted to get in shape," she says. "Working out rejuvenates me mentally and helps me cope."

With baby number four on the way, Maria is back to exercising regularly. But her kids remain her top priority. "I devote each and every day to them," she says. "Connor's illness has taught us to enjoy our time together as a family."

W I N N I N G   A C T I O N

Eat what you want—in moderation. *When trying to slim down, many women deny themselves certain "bad" foods and chastise themselves if they indulge. That's not a realistic or healthy approach to weight loss. If you love chocolate, telling yourself that you can never have it again will only make you want it more. You run the risk of an all-out binge that can permanently derail your weight-loss efforts.*

As long as you eat healthfully most of the time, you can afford periodic splurges. Just keep your portions sen-

sible. If you're hungry for ice cream, for example, don't sit down with a spoon and a half-gallon of your favorite flavor. Scoop a serving into a bowl—and enjoy!

THIS MOM THINKS DIFFERENTLY ABOUT EXERCISE

Melanie Neubelt didn't have a problem shedding her postpregnancy pounds, not even after delivering quadruplets. But she did feel out of shape. As much as she wanted to trim and tone her body, she wasn't interested in the usual activities, such as running, cycling, and strength training. Instead, she charted her own fitness course.

After 3 years of trying to start a family, Melanie and her husband were ecstatic to learn that she was expecting quadruplets. She gained just 40 pounds before delivering Gabrielle, Heidi, Max, and Ethan in January 1995. "My doctors weren't overly concerned, since my babies were growing as they should," she explains. "They arrived 7 weeks prematurely, which is excellent for quads!"

For Melanie's part, she lost all her baby fat within 4 to 6 weeks of delivery. Even though she had returned to her prepregnancy weight—135 pounds on her 5-foot-6 frame—Melanie remembers feeling heavy and uncomfortable. "I probably wasn't overweight by doctors' standards," she says. "But when I whenever I sat down, I felt like I had a sore bottom. It was all flab and no muscle."

Still, with four babies to care for, Melanie hardly even thought about exercising. "Even if I'd had the time, I would have felt guilty about leaving the kids to go work out," she says. "Besides, I had been very inactive during my pregnancy, and I wasn't even sure how to begin getting fit."

When the quads were still less than 2 years old, Melanie became pregnant again. Baby Dominique arrived in January 1997, and within a matter of weeks, her mom had shed all 25 to 30 of her postpregnancy pounds. "But I felt more out of shape than ever," says Melanie.

Two years later, counting down to her 40th birthday, Melanie decided that she couldn't wait any longer to get in shape. "At my age, I can't just let my body go," she says. "I may never get it back!"

To keep her motivation high, Melanie carefully crafted her fitness routine around activities that she thought she might enjoy. She joined a tennis league based near her Little Silver, New Jersey, home, so she could perfect her backhand while building her strength and endurance. And she signed up for jazz dance classes, since she had enjoyed dancing before her pregnancies.

Melanie also made some dietary changes, cutting back on junk food and eating more veggies. But she credits her unique fitness routine with slimming and shaping her body, which has more of the muscle tone and definition that she wanted. "I've even lost 10 pounds!" she says.

Melanie has no intention of giving up her workouts. She enjoys the opportunity to get out and mingle with other people. "Since I pay to participate and funds are tight, I have extra motivation to go," she says. "And the kids love to tag along!"

WINNING ACTION

Expand your fitness horizons. *Anything that gets you moving can work your muscles, burn calories, and help you shed those postpregnancy pounds. So don't feel obligated to stick with a conventional activity such as walking, running, or cycling (though if you enjoy one of* *these, by all means go for it). Use your imagination! Sign up for a dance or martial arts class, take up ice-skating or rock climbing, or join a local volleyball or golf league. You may even be able to find an activity in which the whole family can participate. Just make sure that it's something <u>you</u> enjoy so that you'll want to stick with it.*

HOME TEAM ROOTS FOR HER WEIGHT-LOSS SUCCESS

Tracy Kenerson wants to be around to enjoy her children for a long, long time. That's why she's determined to shed the 30 pounds of baby fat still lingering from her four pregnancies.

Actually, Tracy's struggle with her weight didn't begin until after her two oldest children—8-year-old Rebecca and 6-year-old R. J.—were born. Like many moms, she had 10 stubborn pounds that she just couldn't seem to lose. But she remained confident that they'd eventually disappear. "Besides, my husband, James, and I wanted more children, so I figured that I'd be gaining more weight anyway," says the 30-year-old New Port Richey, Florida, resident.

Because the first two pregnancies had gone so smoothly, the Kenersons never expected to have trouble conceiving for a third time. But they did. "The more time that passed, the more depressed I became," Tracy recalls. "I started overeating, which I had never done before."

Several years after R. J.'s arrival, the Kenersons finally got the news that they had been waiting for: Tracy was pregnant again. At that point, she weighed 170 pounds—50 more than before her pregnancies. She gained another 50 pounds before delivering son Dillon in January 1998.

Tracy managed to shed 50 pounds before becoming pregnant for a fourth time. This time she gained 50 pounds, then lost 20. After delivering daughter Jamie in February 2000, Tracy's weight stabilized at 220.

At 5 feet 4, Tracy worried about the extra pounds, and not just because of her appearance. "I wanted to see my children grow up and start families of their own," she says. "Because of them, I didn't want to take any unnecessary chances with my health. I didn't want to put myself at risk for heart disease or some other obesity-related medical problem."

So shortly after giving birth to Jamie, Tracy joined Weight Watchers and began following its POINTS system, which assigns points to various foods based on their nutritional value. Tracy can consume a certain number of points each day. "I follow a plan that's designed especially for breastfeeding moms, to ensure that the babies get enough nutrients," she says. "I eat lots of fruits and vegetables, and I drink between 80 and 120 ounces of water per day, plus two glasses of milk."

To further support her weight-loss efforts, Tracy also started exercising regularly. "My children and I walk 3 miles a day, and I practice Tae-Bo every other day," she says. "If I don't feel like walking, the kids make sure that we do: 'Mommy, when are we going for our walk? We're going now, aren't we, Mommy?' You get the picture."

By eating healthfully and exercising regularly, Tracy shed 61 pounds in 9 months. Her goal is to reach 140—20 pounds more than her prepregnancy weight, but appropriate for her 5-foot-4 frame. "It's become something of a family effort," she says. "My kids are helping me to slim down, and in return, I'm teaching them the basics of a healthy lifestyle. I want to be a good example for them."

WINNING ACTION

Turn to your children for inspiration. *Sometimes the promise of a slimmer, shapelier physique may not be enough to persuade you to stick with your postpartum weight-loss plan. When you feel your motivation slipping, remind yourself of the other benefits of shedding those extra pounds. You can reduce your risk of heart disease, type 2 diabetes, and certain kinds of cancer. You can lower your cholesterol and blood pressure levels. You can protect yourself against arthritis. With benefits like these, you'll be able to maintain a healthy, active, vital presence in your children's lives for years to come. You'll be around to celebrate every milestone with them. Use them as your motivation to pursue your weight-loss goals.*

SHE LOST WEIGHT BY PRIORITIZING HER DINNER PLATE

If you were to add together the weight gain from Roberta Herron's two pregnancies—one with twins—you'd see that she picked up enough poundage to almost double her body weight. Yet each time she slimmed down to her prepregnancy figure. She adopted the usual lifestyle changes, making sure to eat healthfully and exercise regularly. But she credits an unusual strategy with giving her an edge on weight-loss success: Rather than reducing the amount of food on her dinner plate, she ate it in a different order.

Roberta didn't always exert such control over her eating habits. In fact, she attributes the weight gain during her first pregnancy—with Julia, who's now age 4—to a pattern of overindulging. "I ate anything that tasted good, and I ate a lot of it," admits Roberta, a 38-year-old Syracuse, New York, resident. She ended up adding 60 extra pounds to her 5-foot-3 frame before Julia was born.

She put on the same amount of weight during her second pregnancy, with twins, Sean and Christopher, who are now 23 months old. "I got heavier faster the second time around," she says. "Just carrying twins is a strain on the body, never mind the extra pounds."

Despite the apparent odds against her, Roberta won her war on baby fat, dropping down to 125, her prepregnancy weight, within a year of each delivery. She did it in part by rethinking her approach to mealtimes. "I didn't actually eliminate anything from my meals," she explains. "But rather than digging into the meat or the potatoes, as I had usually done, I started with the vegetables. And I finished them off before moving on to another food."

By filling up on veggies first, Roberta had less room for fatty and starchy foods like meat and potatoes. And eating smaller amounts of those foods gave her a head start on slimming down successfully.

Once she started losing, Roberta kept track of her weight and measurements in a journal. "My journal became a fabulous incentive for me," she says. "I could see when I had reached a plateau in terms of pounds and inches lost, so I could make adjustments in my eating habits or exercise routine."

Since returning to her prepregnancy weight for a second time, Roberta has remained as slim and shapely as ever. That won't change, she says, as long as she remembers her priorities at the dinner table.

Eat your veggies first, then move on to the entrée. *By moving vegetables (and fruits) to the top of the food chain, you're starting your meal with an abundance of vitamins, minerals, and other key nutrients. You can still enjoy the other stuff on your plate, but more than likely, you'll eat less than you would have otherwise. It's an effective means of controlling calorie and fat intake as well as portion size. Yet it doesn't leave you feeling deprived. It's a fabulous strategy for melting away those postpregnancy pounds.*

THIS MOM IS FIRED UP FOR FITNESS

Firefighting is among the most demanding and dangerous of occupations, requiring tremendous physical strength and endurance. Cindy Fagiano should know: The 41-year-old Chicago native has been battling blazes for 13½ years and through two pregnancies.

Cindy knows all too well the struggles of staying fit, especially once kids enter the picture. But she has to find time to work out. Otherwise, she might not be able to do her job. "I just want to be a good firefighter," she says. "That's my motivation to stay in shape."

Even while she was pregnant with her children—Rocco, who's now 7, and Carissa, who's 4—Cindy's commitment to fitness never faltered. She went on medical leave 2 months into each pregnancy but continued exercising until the day before delivery. As a result, she gained just 30 pounds during both of her pregnancies, and each time, the weight came off within a matter of months. She resumed her firefighting duties when her babies were 3½ months old—and she was as trim and fit as ever.

Cindy never doubted that she'd be able to slim down after having her kids. "Taking care of my body is a way of life for me," she explains. "I've never let myself get out of shape, and I never will."

Cindy remains very active, doing some form of aerobic exercise—step aerobics, stairclimbing, biking, swimming, or walking—five times a week. On those days when she teaches two or three aerobics classes, that counts as her workout.

Today, Cindy carries 168 pounds on her 5-foot-10 body, just 6 pounds more than before her first pregnancy. You might say that her baby fat has gone up in smoke.

WINNING ACTION

Volunteer for an activity that demands physical fitness.
In many communities, firefighting is a volunteer activity. Even if battling blazes doesn't appeal to you, you can likely find other organizations that are always in need of helping hands. Choose an activity that suits your personal preferences. Perhaps you can coach your child's soccer team, or sign up for your church's roadside cleanup crews, or help clear hiking trails through a local park. The possibilities are endless. You'll feel good about helping others—and in the process, you'll be burning calories and building muscle to melt away those post-pregnancy pounds.

MOTHER OF SEXTUPLETS RECLAIMS HER PREPREGNANCY FIGURE

Chris Ann and Christopher Collins very much wanted a large family. But the Kingswood, Texas, couple didn't expect to have one all at once! That's exactly what happened when Chris became pregnant with sextuplets.

After trying to conceive for 12 long years, the Collinses were ecstatic when they learned that Chris was expecting their first child. Their son JonChristopher arrived in June 1997. Just 11 months later, Chris became pregnant again. This time, she was carrying not just one baby but six. "Even though I had been taking fertility drugs, my husband and I were shocked," she recalls. "Imagine—we had seven kids in 17 months!"

Almost immediately, Chris was put on bed rest by her doctor, who expressed concern about the risks associated with carrying six babies at once. Chris worried that such a long period of inactivity would cause her to blow up like a balloon.

But that didn't happen. Instead, Chris developed such severe nausea that she couldn't keep down any food at all. "As the babies grew, my stomach got too crowded," she explains. "Then my doctor worried that I wasn't gaining enough weight."

By her 18th week, Chris looked as if she were in her ninth month. She had to be hospitalized for 2 months before giving birth to her babies. Christopher arrived first, in October 1998—25 days before his siblings, Jeremiah, Rebekah, Noah, Hannah, and Faith. As large as she had been, Chris was left with only 35 extra pounds.

The Collins family was quickly swept up in a swirl of national media attention, a situation that both frustrated and motivated Chris. "On the one hand, I resented the loss of privacy," she says.

"On the other hand, I wanted to go on TV looking good. I know how critical some people can be."

She certainly didn't need to worry about getting enough exercise. From the time she got up in the morning until the time she went to bed, Chris was constantly on the go. "I can't even guess how many miles I put in just running around the house," she laughs. While she didn't go on a diet, she did become more conscientious about her food choices. "No soda, no chips, no other junk food," she says. "I try to eat healthier snacks, like yogurt. And I take a multivitamin every day."

These strategies were enough to drop Chris—who's 5 feet 6—to 125 pounds, her prepregnancy weight. Perhaps just as amazing, she reached that mark within a month of delivering the sextuplets.

To this day, people who meet Chris for the first time can't believe that she's a mother of seven, let alone a set of sextuplets. "Usually they ask me, 'You've had *how many* kids?'" she laughs. "I guess they're expecting me to be overweight and out of shape."

The stunned reactions of others inspire Chris, who's now 34, to maintain her trim physique. "I probably could get by with the extra pounds, because people would just say, 'Well, look how many kids she's had,'" she says. "But I'd rather feel good about myself."

WINNING ACTION

Make minor adjustments to score major results. *Whether you've had one baby or six, you don't need to make sweeping changes in your lifestyle in order to lose postpregnancy pounds. Nor would you want to—especially not when so many other aspects of your life have been turned upside down with the arrival of a newborn. Instead, look for ways to tweak your eating habits and* *exercise program. For instance, switch from low-fat milk to fat-free; top your morning toast with fruit spread instead of butter or margarine; extend your regular workout by 5 minutes. These sorts of changes can really add up in terms of taking off the baby fat. And they're so innocuous that they'll be easy to stick with.*

GUILT-FREE MEALS KEEP THIS MOM TRIM

Like every mom-to-be, Christine Okoniewski expected to gain weight during her first pregnancy. But she had no idea just how much she had gained until she saw herself in a photo taken at a Labor Day picnic about a year after daughter Meghan, now age 4, was born.

"When I looked at the photo, I thought, 'Wow, am I really that big? Are my arms really that fat?'" recalls Christine, a 36-year-old homemaker from Newark, Delaware. "I joined Weight Watchers the very next Thursday."

In fact, while carrying Meghan, Christine had added about 25 pounds to her 5-foot-4, 155-pound body. By the time she joined Weight Watchers—14 months after giving birth—she had lost just 12 pounds.

"Weight Watchers provided the structure and support that I needed to slim down," Christine explains. "It also taught me the importance of balanced eating and regular exercise." Most important, it enabled her to lose the rest of her baby fat—and then some. By Meghan's second birthday, Christine was down to 138 pounds.

She maintained her weight for a year before becoming pregnant again.

After giving birth to baby Jack in July 1999, Christine had another 27 pounds to lose. She went back to Weight Watchers because it had worked so well after her first pregnancy. But this time, she came up with her own strategy for maintaining her motivation until she reached her prepregnancy weight.

From Sunday through Thursday, Christine followed the Weight Watchers eating plan to the letter. But on Friday and Saturday, she rewarded herself with a "free eating night," when she could have whatever she wanted for dinner. "I had to let myself live a little," she explains. "The freedom that I enjoyed for those two meals encouraged me to eat healthier the rest of the week."

Her strategy worked wonders. Within 9 months of delivering Jack, Christine had reached 142 pounds—just 4 pounds shy of her prepregnancy weight. Even when she reaches her goal, she has no intention of letting her eating-and-exercise plan slide. "I understand that I have to eat healthfully and exercise regularly for the rest of my life," she says. "That's the only way that I'll maintain my weight."

WINNING ACTION

Allow yourself to splurge for one meal each week. *Even the most inspired eating plan can seem utterly unsatisfying if it completely disregards your favorite foods. That's why you should make room for at least one "treat meal" in your week. That flexibility just might give you incentive to eat better at other meals—and an edge in achieving your weight-loss goal.*

SHE HAS MADE EXERCISE A FAMILY AFFAIR

In June 2000, Catherine Beisel became a mom for the third time. Though the pregnancy left her carrying 45 extra pounds, she was confident that the weight would soon disappear. After all, she had won the baby-fat war twice before, losing a total of 80 pounds. This time, as the last, she would have her kids to help her slim down.

Catherine, a 35-year-old Bayport, New York, resident, had built a lifestyle around eating healthfully and exercising regularly. And it showed: When she became pregnant with her first child in 1993, she weighed 135 pounds—appropriate for her 5-foot-7 frame. She gained 40 pounds before son Jack was born.

"As it happened, my best friend was getting married just 2 months after I delivered Jack, and I was in the bridal party," Catherine recalls. "I didn't want to look bad wearing the long, sleek bridesmaid gown. That motivated me to slim down as quickly as possible."

Six weeks postpartum, Catherine began taking step aerobics classes at a local gym. She lost nearly 30 pounds by her friend's wedding day. The rest of her baby fat disappeared within the year, as she added walking to her exercise routine and shrank her portion sizes at meals.

Two years later, in 1996, Catherine became pregnant with her second child. She had another boy, Eric—and gained another 40 pounds. With two tots to care for, Catherine couldn't swing going back to the gym. Still, she was eager to resume her fitness program and lose her postpregnancy pounds.

Then one day Catherine's husband brought home a child's seat to attach to an old bicycle that had been lying in the Beisels' garage. Soon enough, Catherine and her 3-year-old were spending their evenings pedaling around their neighborhood, while her husband stayed home with the baby.

"We're just a short ride from the beach, so we got to enjoy lots of beautiful scenery," Catherine says. "Plus, I got to spend some quality time with my son."

As the baby got older, Catherine altered her exercise routine to include him as well, pushing him in a stroller while her older son rode his plastic motorcycle. "Both boys loved going to the marina to watch the boats come in," she says. "They motivated me to be active." Within a year of her younger son's arrival, she shed every pound of baby fat and was back to her prepregnancy weight of 135.

Those evening outings remained a family ritual for the Beisels. Five nights a week, they'd eat dinner, then walk or ride down to the marina. "It gave the boys a chance to wind down, so they'd be ready for bed by the time we got home," Catherine says. "More important, we were spending time together as a family."

Unfortunately, Catherine's third pregnancy forced her to cut back on her physical activity. She was sick through her first trimester, and the cold winter temperatures kept her indoors through her second trimester. After the birth of her third child, daughter Charlotte, in June 2000, she couldn't wait to start exercising again.

It wasn't just the 45 postpregnancy pounds that motivated Catherine. "I miss the exercise, and I miss the time with my family," she says. "I can't wait to get back on my bike and head for the beach!" With that kind of enthusiasm, Catherine is certain to achieve another victory in the baby-fat war.

WINNING ACTION

Skip the sitter and let your kids work out with you. *No matter what your child's age, you can find a way to in-*

corporate the youngster into your fitness program. Doing so has benefits for both of you. Your child can persuade you to go for a walk or bike ride, even when you may not want to. In return, you can set a good example for your child by leading an active lifestyle. Plus, the two of you get to spend some time together, so you stay connected with each other.

You might even try some of the activities that your child loves. Play tag or Frisbee. Mix a little hopping and skipping into your walks. You'll get a good workout, and you'll have fun to boot!

MOTHER OF FIVE STAYS FIT BY KEEPING UP WITH HER KIDS

Robbin Forristall weighs just 5 pounds more at age 37 than at age 21. That fact alone is impressive. It's downright amazing when you consider that the Ashland, Ohio, native has five children, including two sets of twins.

How does she keep herself so trim? Even Robbin admits that she doesn't have the healthiest lifestyle. The self-proclaimed Pepsi junkie isn't all that careful about her diet. She's not big on exercise either.

But Robbin is getting plenty of physical activity, even though she's not working out in a gym. She figures that just chasing after her kids keeps her fit. "I'm constantly on the go," she says. "I don't have time to sit around and get fat!"

Even before she started a family, Robbin led a very active

lifestyle. And it showed: She carried just 115 pounds on her 5-foot-7 body. She delivered the oldest twins, Joseph and Julius, in February 1984, followed by Jarrett in March 1998. Each time she slimmed down soon after delivery. All told, she lost 124 pounds of baby fat—plus 3 extra for good measure.

Robbin's success at slimming down continued after her third pregnancy with the youngest twins, Joshua and Jenna, who are just 5 months old. This time around she lost 48 pounds of baby fat, which put her at a healthy 120.

With two teens, a preschooler, and two infants to care for, Robbin seems destined to maintain her weight with ease. "Just chasing after a 2-year-old is a workout," she says. "When the babies get older, they'll really keep me busy!"

Robbin isn't just keeping up with her kids, she's cleaning up after them, too. She estimates that she goes up and down her basement stairs an average of 25 times a day, making trips to the laundry room, the playroom, and the oldest twins' bedrooms. "It's sort of like a stairclimbing machine, but without the motor," she says.

As tired as she feels some days—"Sleep? What is that?" she jokes—Robbin wouldn't trade her hectic lifestyle for the world. She loves her kids, and she's grateful to them for keeping her on her toes. They're the reason that she looks as good today as she did 16 years ago.

WINNING ACTION

Keep up with your kids. *As your family grows, you may have less time for a formal fitness program. But that doesn't mean you can't stay active. Just running after your kids can give you a good workout, especially if you have a toddler. Don't overlook the value of this very* *basic form of exercise. It helps you slim down, and in the process, it gets your children hooked on physical activity from an early age. Together, you'll discover that fitness can be fun.*

THIS MOM HOPES HISTORY WILL REPEAT ITSELF

Carol Barone had 50 good reasons for wanting to manage her weight gain through her two pregnancies. The Lagrangeville, New York, resident had lost that many pounds in the early 1990s. While she always dreamed of becoming a mom, she was determined not to wrestle with her weight again.

Carol and her husband, Carl, planned to start a family soon after they got married in November 1995. Their dreams were realized not quite a year later, when Carol learned that she was pregnant.

Having already gained the infamous "honeymoon 10," Carol knew that she needed to be extravigilant to avoid gaining too many pregnancy pounds. "I watched everything that I ate," she says. "I didn't buy into the notion that I could eat more just because I was pregnant." For exercise, she just continued the walking routine that she had started before becoming pregnant.

Carol held her prenatal weight gain to 32 pounds, appropriate for a woman of her size—5 feet, 132 pounds. She gave birth to son Connor in May 1997, then lost all but 10 pounds of baby fat over the next 3 months or so. Those 10 were still hanging on more than a year and a half later, when Carol found out that she was expecting again.

"The second time, I really didn't make any dietary changes, mainly because I was just too tired to eat," Carol says. "Between running after Connor and taking care of the house, I had my hands full."

Being pregnant through the summer had an effect, too. "It was so hot that I just stopped gaining weight around my seventh month," Carol recalls. "My doctor said that as long as my vital signs, like my blood pressure, were okay, he didn't see a reason to be concerned."

By the time daughter Caylea arrived in October 1999, Carol had gained just 22 pounds. "And I lost all of them within the first month after delivery," she says.

With all of the baby fat from her second pregnancy gone, Carol, who's now 43, has a new goal: to shed the 10 pounds left over from her first pregnancy, plus her "honeymoon 10." When she succeeds, she'll be back to her wedding-day weight of 122.

"My husband gained the 'honeymoon 10,' too, so now we're both trying to slim down," Carol says. "We're walking together, as often as possible. And we're eating less fat than we used to."

Whenever she feels her motivation sagging, Carol reminds herself of the 50 pounds that she shed a decade ago. "It keeps me on track," she says. "It convinces me that I can reach my goal again."

WINNING ACTION

Draw inspiration from prior weight-loss success. *If you've struggled with your weight, you may be especially concerned about the extra pounds that pregnancy can leave behind. Instead of worrying, remind yourself of your past weight-loss success. Use it to build your confidence, to prove to yourself that you know how to* *win the fat war. Think about the strategies that worked previously and whether they might be helpful during and after your pregnancy. Remember: You've done it before, so you can do it again!*

SHE FINDS STRENGTH IN NUMBERS

After being pregnant three times in 4 years, Julie Lane barely recognized her formerly svelte body underneath 100 pounds of baby fat. Now, however, she's just 13 pounds away from achieving her goal weight. She has her Slim Sisters—her cyberspace weight-loss team—to thank for her success.

Julie, a 25-year-old Arlington, Texas, resident, discovered the power of online support groups after her first child, Bryan, was stillborn in December 1996. Grief-stricken, she turned to food for comfort. "I started eating anything and everything," she recalls. "I'd get sad, so I'd eat. Then I'd get mad at myself for eating. It was a rollercoaster ride."

Already carrying 75 extra pounds from her pregnancy, Julie found herself gaining even more. That only added to her misery. "Because I kept getting heavier, people assumed that I was pregnant," she says. "It upset me so much that I became desperate to slim down."

Julie resorted to what she describes as starvation dieting to get rid of the excess weight. She managed to lose 25 pounds before learning that she was once again expecting, 3 months after her first pregnancy.

Buoyed by the news of pending motherhood, Julie realized that bingeing on food and then starving herself was not helping her to cope with her son Bryan's death. She decided to use the Internet to seek out message boards for families dealing with similar tragedies. Through the support she found online, Julie began to heal.

When their son Brett arrived in December 1997, the Lanes were jubilant. But Julie's joy soon gave way to concern when she realized that she had added another 30 pounds to her 5-foot-5 frame. Once a slim and shapely 120, she was now inching toward the 200 mark.

But Julie scarcely had time to consider her weight-loss options before becoming pregnant for a third time. When her daughter, Blair, was born in September 1999, Julie weighed 229 pounds. "I felt like I was trapped in my own body," she recalls.

In an effort to slim down, Julie began following a high-protein diet. She also practiced Tae-Bo 3 days a week. "I managed to lose 43 pounds, but I ran out of steam by the end of November," she says.

Once again, Julie resorted to the quick-fix weight-loss schemes. "I tried a 'metabolic enhancement' product, but it gave me mood swings and jitters," she says. "When I went off it, I cried for 3 days."

Julie finally accepted the fact that she wouldn't find a "magic pill" to help her slim down. She'd have to do it the healthy way, through nutritious eating and regular exercise.

As a stay-at-home mom with a toddler and an infant in her care, Julie didn't have the time or money to join a conventional weight-loss program. So she consulted books like *Body for Life* by Bill Phillips and Michael D'Orso, gleaning as much information as she could to formulate her own eating-and-exercise plan.

Julie knew that she needed help to jump-start her weight-loss efforts. Remembering how online support had given her strength and hope after her son's death, she decided to turn to cyberspace once again.

Searching the Internet, Julie discovered a Web site called

ParentsPlace.com, with a message board tailored to postpregnancy weight loss. She decided to post a message expressing her interest in joining a support group. Soon after, she was assigned to a team with five other women—four from the United States and one from Canada. All had the same objective: to get rid of their baby fat.

"We voted on our team name, and Slim Sisters won," Julie says. "Then I volunteered to design a Web site just for us, where we could keep track of our weekly weigh-ins and brag about our accomplishments." Through the site, the women have formed a real bond. "We cheer when one of us reaches a goal, and we sympathize when one of us breaks down and has a piece of apple pie," Julie says. "We've gotten to know each other really well, and we're having lots of fun."

Since joining the Slim Sisters in December 1999, Julie has lost another 53 pounds. She's just 13 pounds away from 120, her prepregnancy weight. "I'm exercising six times a week, alternating aerobic workouts with weight training, and I'm making healthful food choices," she says. "I've had moments where I've wanted to give in to a craving or to skip a workout. But then I think of the Slim Sisters, and they help me stay on track. I couldn't do it without them."

WINNING ACTION

Seek out support in cyberspace. *If you find yourself lacking the inspiration and motivation to stick with your weight-loss program, remember that you don't have to go it alone. The Internet is teeming with Web sites and message boards for weight loss (including, of course, our very own Prevention.com). Some, like ParentsPlace.com, are specifically for new moms. You'll meet other women just like you, who want to take off their postpregnancy pounds. You'll cheer each other when you achieve* *seemingly small victories, and pump each other up when your spirits are flagging. If you choose, you can remain anonymous. And you can log on at any time—a bonus for moms who are pressed for time. "What I like is that we're not always talking about diet and exercise," Julie says. "We share parenting advice, too."*

SHE'S EATING BETTER FOR HER KIDS' SAKE

In hindsight, Kristy Corino realizes how lucky she was. Before becoming pregnant with twins, she managed to maintain her 5-foot-2 frame at a slim 101 pounds, despite an insatiable sweet tooth that she indulged freely. Now that she's a mom, she's more conscientious about her eating habits. After all, she has to set a good example for her kids.

Kristy, a 37-year-old Blue Bell, Pennsylvania, resident, admits that she wasn't always so concerned about what she ate. "Before the babies, I would have nothing but junk for lunch," she remembers. "The sweets definitely outweighed the fruits and vegetables." And every afternoon around 3 o'clock, she helped herself to a candy bar—for energy, she says.

With news of her impending motherhood, Kristy did make an effort to clean up her eating habits. But she didn't get really serious about it until after the twins, Brad and Julianna, arrived in July 1998. While Kristy had gained 43 pounds during her pregnancy, she lost all but 3 of those pounds within 5 days of her delivery. "But I expected to have a hard time keeping off the weight, because my body had changed," she explains.

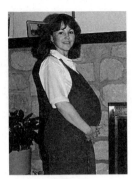

9 months pregnant

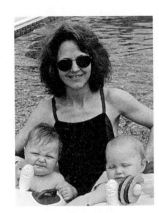

1 year after delivery

Staying slim wasn't Kristy's only motivation for eating better. She also felt a responsibility toward her children. "I want them to have good eating habits," she explains. "But how can I expect them to choose fruits and vegetables when they see me filling up on junk food? I need to be a good role model for them."

Realizing her obligation to her kids, Kristy has drastically cut back on her junk food consumption. These days, breakfast usually consists of cereal and fruit; for lunch, she eats yogurt with wheat germ and fruit. She no longer takes an afternoon candy-bar break, and at family meals, she serves fresh fruit instead of ice cream for dessert. "I do have a dish of ice cream at night after the kids have gone to bed," she says. "It's the one food I just can't give up."

Thanks to Kristy's new and improved eating habits, her weight has held steady at 104 pounds ever since she gave birth to her babies. The positive influence of her healthy food choices will surely become more apparent as the twins get older. "I can see it already," she says. "Half the time when I offer them cookies, they reply, 'No thanks, Mommy!' They really like their fruits and vegetables!"

WINNING ACTION

See yourself through your children's eyes. Your kids learn many of their behaviors, especially their eating habits, just by watching you. So you can't very well fill up on junk food or skip breakfast or order pizza for dinner five nights a week without those choices having some effect on your children—not to mention your waistline. Think of the image that you present to your kids when you eat unhealthfully. That may be enough to keep your eating habits in line—and to make those extra pounds disappear.

WANT TO SLIM DOWN? THIS MOM SAYS, "JOIN THE CLUB!"

When Debby Gage wanted to shed the 7 to 8 pounds left behind by her second pregnancy, she joined a gym. That may not seem like the most revolutionary weight-loss strategy. But the fact is, many new moms say that they don't have the time or the energy to work out. Debby found that her gym's flexible schedule and varied activities helped her stick with her fitness routine and eventually drop down to her prepregnancy weight.

Debby had every reason to want to slim down quickly. She worried that because of her age, 35, she'd have a hard time getting rid of the extra pounds. And she certainly didn't want them to become permanent.

To her advantage, she had prior weight-loss success on her side. During her pregnancy with her son, now 6, she added 21 pounds to her petite 4-foot-10 frame. She lost all but 3 of those pounds within 9 to 10 months, thanks to a combination of eating healthfully, walking regularly, and working out on a NordicTrack machine.

But when she became pregnant with her daughter, now 3, Debby struggled almost from the start. "With my son, I had taken a special prenatal fitness class, and I had a videotape of the class that I intended to use again," she explains. "But I lent the tape to someone else, and I never got it back."

As for her eating habits, while she ate very well—lots of grains, fruits, and vegetables—she also nibbled quite a bit. "My snacking has gotten a lot worse over the years," she admits.

By then, Debby and her family were living in a new home in Merrick, New York. It just happened to have a swimming pool. To control her prenatal weight gain, Debby began fitness-swimming regularly. "I worked my way up to ½ mile three times a week," she says. "In fact, I did laps the day that I went into labor."

Her routine must have helped, because she ended up gaining a healthy 25 pounds through her second pregnancy. But she knew that she'd have a harder time slimming down. "First, I was older," she says. "Second, I had a toddler and an infant to care for."

In a similar situation, other women might have put their exercise programs on permanent hold. But Debby knew that she had to stay active in order to lose those extra pounds. After much thought, she decided to join a nearby gym. "I figured that if I had someplace to go, and specific days and times to be there, I would work out more," she says. "I certainly wasn't working out enough on my own."

Debby went to the gym 3 days a week, usually while her son was in school and her daughter was with her babysitter. Each of her sessions combined 45 minutes of aerobic exercise—usually running or walking—with 15 to 20 minutes of strength training and toning. "If

I got bored, I'd use one of the elliptical machines, or I'd take a class," she says. "I could do what I wanted, when I wanted. That was great motivation."

Over the course of 5 months, Debby lost the last of her baby fat. Since then, her weight has stabilized at 96 pounds. "I weigh more than before both my pregnancies, but I suspect that's because I have more muscle mass now," she says.

Now age 35, Debby continues to go to the gym to work out. "I do try to fit in some outdoor activities with the kids," she says. "I'll go for a walk with my daughter in her stroller, or I'll ride bikes with my son. But I still count on the gym for staying fit."

WINNING ACTION

Get in with the gym crowd. *You may think of health clubs as havens for muscle-bound guys and spandex-clad girls, certainly not the sort of place where a mom with a few extra pounds would feel comfortable exercising. If that's your perspective, then you really owe it to yourself to check out your local fitness facilities. They offer all kinds of activities and classes, with flexible hours and schedules that allow you to come and go as you please. Virtually all of them have personal trainers right on staff, and many offer on-site child care. The fact that you must pay for your membership may serve as an additional motivator: You'll want to be sure to get your money's worth.*

SLIMMING DOWN WAS WORTH THE "WEIGHT"

After shedding the 20-plus pounds of baby fat left behind by each of her two pregnancies, Rose Perkins wanted to make sure that the weight didn't come back. So she added strength training to her fitness regimen. Has it helped? Well, consider this: She wears the same size now as before she had her kids!

Fitness has been part of Rose's life for as long as she can remember. The 35-year-old Lancaster, Massachusetts, native was an avid figure skater through most of her childhood. Even as she grew up, she never slowed down, moving from skating to aerobics and step aerobics classes. Her focus on fitness encouraged her to eat healthfully, too. "I can't say that I ever went on a diet," she says. "I paid attention to my food choices, but I tried not to deny myself anything."

By the time she became pregnant with her oldest daughter, Kayla, now age 7, Rose was working for a company with an on-site fitness center. "I would go there every day on my lunch hour," she says. "I exercised right up to delivery with both of my kids."

Rose gained 23 pounds with Kayla and 22 pounds with her youngest daughter, Shannon, age 5. Both times she lost the weight by her 6-week postpartum checkup. "I believe that breastfeeding played a big part in my slimming down so quickly," she says. "But staying active helped, too."

Even though she returned to her prepregnancy weight—118 pounds on her 5-foot-6½-inch body—Rose never lost her commitment to fitness. On the contrary, she began toying with the idea of adding strength training to her exercise program. "I knew that the extra muscle would burn extra calories, which would help maintain my weight," she says. "Besides, strength training would protect my bones against osteoporosis, which affected my grandmother."

But like many women, Rose also had some reservations about lifting weights. "I didn't want to get big and bulky," she explains. "But our on-site fitness trainer, Norma Fay, put my fears to rest. She emphasized the importance of being strong to avoid injuries in everyday life—from lifting kids or moving furniture, for example. And she reminded us that with the increased muscle mass, we could eat more and not worry about it. Our bodies would burn the extra calories, even while we're at rest."

With Norma's guidance, Rose began strength training two or three times a week, using a combination of free weights and weight machines. She continued her aerobic workouts at least three times a week, switching between aerobics classes and cardiovascular machines, such as the stairclimber and the treadmill.

Rose has maintained this routine since 1995, after the birth of her second daughter. Today, she weighs 122—which is 4 pounds more than before her pregnancy. Because her clothing size hasn't changed, she attributes the weight gain to her increased muscle mass.

Rose started strength training to stay slim and protect her bones. It has done that—and more. "It has made me stronger and given my body more definition. I don't feel like a weakling anymore," she says. "I don't want to become fragile later in life. I want to stay active for as long as possible."

WINNING ACTION

Pick up some weights to put away the baby fat. *Strength training builds muscle mass. And extra muscle means greater calorie burn, even when you're at rest, so baby fat will be gone before you know it. You don't want to* *start lifting too soon after delivery, as the exertion can be hard on a postpartum body. Be sure to get your doctor's okay first, and work with a personal trainer at least until you learn proper technique. Many experts recommend lifting two or three times a week, alternating between strength training and aerobic workouts.*

PICTURE THIS: 34 POUNDS OF BABY FAT—GONE

Linda Sundlin wasn't asking for much. The Los Angeles resident just wanted to look good in a swimsuit again. But after a 4-year struggle against baby fat, she feared that her prepregnancy figure had vanished for good.

Linda had been at odds with her weight ever since delivering her first child, Henni, in 1991. Her once-svelte physique—5 feet 7, 145 pounds—grew heavier and softer, despite Linda's best efforts to stay in shape. While she lost 20 pounds of baby fat within a month of giving birth, she regained 25 over the next 2 years. She reached her top weight, 200 pounds, while pregnant with her second child.

After giving birth to baby Tanner in May 1995, Linda unwittingly repeated the pattern from her first pregnancy. She lost 35 pounds in 6 months, then regained 30 over the next 2 years. "I tried just about every diet and every form of exercise imaginable," she recalls. "I was about to resign myself to the fact that I'd never be slim again."

In a last-ditch effort to shed her baby fat, Linda consulted a personal trainer, who advised her to keep a food journal. "I wrote down everything that I ate, which helped me to keep tabs on my fat and sugar intakes," she says. "It also guided me toward healthier food choices."

Not long after she started her food journal, Linda was flipping through a swimsuit catalog when a certain photo caught her eye. The woman had a figure much like Linda's before her pregnancies—sleek and strong, though not model-thin. "I had looked like that once, and I wanted to look like that again," Linda explains. So she tore out the photo and pasted it into her journal.

Now whenever she wants to document her food intake, Linda must look at the image of her slender alter ego. It inspires her to remain steadfast in her pursuit of her weight-loss goals. After watching her weight seesaw for several years, she dropped 34 pounds in just 1 year. At age 44, she's just 11 pounds away from her goal weight—and her swimsuit.

WINNING ACTION

Find a photo that fits your weight-loss goals. *If you're like most women, you're slimming down by aiming for a particular number on the bathroom scale. You can make that number seem more real and attainable by associating it with a particular visual image. Round up a photo of yourself at your ideal weight. If you don't have one, browse through some magazines or catalogs until you find a photo of someone who closely matches your own body type. But be realistic: Comparing your body with the airbrushed image of a supermodel is only going to frustrate you in the long run. Instead, choose a photo of someone who seems fit and healthy. Then post that image where you can see it on a regular basis. Use it as your motivation to shed that baby fat.*

IN THE BATTLE AGAINST BABY FAT, THIS MOM SCORES BIG

Elicia Nolan has redefined the term *soccer mom*. While other parents watch the game from the sidelines, she's actually playing it. She credits the sport with helping her to shape up after both of her pregnancies—and to lose 70 postpregnancy pounds.

Elicia first set foot on a soccer field when she was an 11-year-old elementary school student playing in a league with her friends. As she got older, she lost interest in the sport. She never expected to be playing again years later, as a 31-year-old mother of two.

But not long after giving birth to son Jerry in September 1996, Elicia was invited by a friend to join an indoor soccer league. "I really didn't want to play, but she convinced me to try it," recalls Elicia, a resident of St. James, New York.

Her friend had good instincts, because once Elicia started playing again, she absolutely loved it. "I was surprised by the competitiveness of the games, and the roughness," she says. "But I could feel myself getting better every time I stepped on the field."

Elicia's team is one of eight in an all-female soccer league. These days, she plays two games—one indoors and one outdoors—almost every week. She did take some time off while pregnant with daughter Catherine, whom she delivered in February 1998. As soon as she felt up to it, she was back on the field, kicking around the ball.

Indeed, soccer did wonders for Elicia's postpregnancy figure. While she gained 30 pounds with Jerry and 40 with Catherine, she lost all of the weight within months of each delivery. She has maintained her 5-foot-6 body at 140 pounds since shortly after Catherine's arrival.

Soccer has produced other changes in Elicia's body as well. In her position as midfielder, she does a lot of running up and down the field. That has dramatically increased her stamina and improved her muscle tone. "I think I'd be fit even if I wasn't playing soccer," she says. "But I definitely wouldn't have the same muscle tone."

For a woman who once showed little interest in soccer, Elicia has certainly become passionate about it. She intends to keep playing for as long as she can. She has already turned the sport into a family affair: She's the coach for Jerry's soccer team.

WINNING ACTION

Let team sports give you a weight-loss edge. *Does the idea of a little friendly competition with a worthy opponent pique your interest? Then you may want to explore team sports as an alternative to conventional fitness activities like walking, running, and cycling. Many communities have recreational athletic leagues for adults in sports like soccer, softball, basketball, and volleyball. Perhaps your workplace or your church sponsors a team. If not, check out your local health clubs and YM/YWCAs for leads. You can experience the thrill of victory while winning the war against baby fat.*

MOTHER OF FOUR WATCHES AS HER WEIGHT DISAPPEARS

Donna McKim knows a thing or two about postpartum weight loss. The Coatesville, Pennsylvania, resident shed close to 200 pounds of baby fat over the course of four pregnancies. She credits her success to a combination of good nutrition, regular exercise, and a little help from Weight Watchers.

Donna first signed up for Weight Watchers at age 21, when she found herself saddled with some unwanted "college pounds." She was so pleased with the results (she shed 33 of those pounds) that she re-enrolled a few years later, after regaining some of the weight. She has been a member ever since.

While Donna values the advice on nutrition and fitness provided through Weight Watchers, she has always been fairly good about eating healthfully and exercising regularly. She stayed in the program because it kept her in line. "That element of accountability in the form of monthly meetings and weigh-ins has always appealed to me," she says.

It certainly seemed to work for her, if her success in shedding her postpregnancy pounds is any indication. Donna stayed in Weight Watchers even while pregnant with her first three children (the program no longer accepts moms-to-be), then went back 6 to 8 weeks after each delivery. She gained a little more weight with each of her babies—from 30 pounds with her oldest daughter, Sarah, who's now 10, to 60 pounds with her youngest son, James, who's just 2. And she admits that the weight hung around longer each time.

"I got a little spoiled with Sarah, because I lost all of the weight by my 6-week postpartum checkup," Donna says. "With each child since, I had more responsibilities, more obligations, and less time for myself. Sometimes I felt like I'd never slim down. But I did."

And how! At age 36, Donna is maintaining her 5-foot-7 figure at a trim 125 pounds. She won her last battle against baby fat in 1999, when she got rid of the few pounds left over from her pregnancy with James. "Even though I'm happy with my weight, I'm still going to Weight Watchers," she says. "I want to be sure that none of those pounds comes back!"

WINNING ACTION

After baby arrives, enlist the aid of the weight-loss professionals. *Weight Watchers is one of many organizations established solely for the purpose of helping people to slim down successfully. You'll find others listed in the yellow pages under the heading "Weight Control Services." The right program can provide the advice and support that you need to achieve your weight-loss goals. Just be wary of those that seem gimmicky or promise improbable results. Check out the programs for yourself, or ask your physician to recommend one.*

CRAVINGS CAN'T SABOTAGE HER WEIGHT-LOSS EFFORTS

Beth Fuller remembers when she could pile her dinner plate with mashed potatoes drowning in gravy and gobble a bowlful of chips and dip every night—without gaining an ounce. That changed when she had her first child. Now a mother of two, she still craves these foods from time to time. But she's come up with some creative ways to satisfy her tastebuds while whittling her waistline.

When Beth became pregnant for the first time, keeping down any food proved to be a challenge. She had hyperemesis, a condition more serious than morning sickness that causes almost-constant vomiting. She spent 7 months of her pregnancy in the hospital to prevent dehydration. "I was connected to a machine that pumped nutrients into my body to feed me and my baby," she says. "I was unable to take anything by mouth, not even a sip of water." During that time, she actually lost weight, dropping from 115 pounds to 98.

After giving birth to daughter Brittany, who's now 6, Beth returned to her old eating habits—and started adding on the pounds. Three years later, her formerly size-4 figure had grown to a size 8, with 140 pounds packed on to her 5-foot-5 frame. "I didn't even realize that I was getting bigger until I saw a photo of myself that had been taken at Christmastime," says the 30-year-old Windsor Heights, West Virginia, resident. "I couldn't believe that was really me."

For the first time in her life, Beth had to watch what she ate. She abandoned her workday lunch runs to fast-food joints and started eating cottage cheese and tuna instead. She gave up dinners of fried pierogies or Mexican fare in favor of baked potatoes and baked chicken. And she stopped helping herself to platefuls of pasta and second helpings of mashed potatoes. "I realized that I was consuming far too many carbohydrates," she explains.

While the rest of her diet shaped up healthfully, Beth still had to contend with some downright persistent cravings. She couldn't just ignore them, so she decided to quiet them with more nutritious alternatives.

When she felt hungry for carbs, for example, Beth cooked up some oatmeal pancakes with tofu and cottage cheese. When she wanted to splurge on pizza, she didn't call Papa John's. Instead, she made her own personal pie using a whole wheat tortilla, diced tomatoes, and a sprinkling of mozzarella cheese.

Satisfying her cravings for chocolate proved the biggest challenge. "I used to eat a big bowl of chocolate ice cream every night," Beth confesses. Now she pacifies her sweet tooth with graham crackers—and once a week, she treats herself to fat-free chocolate pudding or chocolate-flavored protein bars.

By rebuilding her diet around healthy substitutions, along with working out regularly, Beth slimmed down to 125 pounds before becoming pregnant for a second time. Despite a mild recurrence of hyperemesis, she managed to stay active 5 days a week throughout this pregnancy, riding a stationary bike, practicing yoga, or walking. She gained just 13 pounds before delivering her son, Brett, by cesarean section in January 2000. Three months later, she was down to 116—a single pound over her goal weight.

Even though she has reclaimed her prepregnancy figure, Beth has no intention of reverting to her old eating habits. Now that she's making healthier food choices, she's feeling better than she has in a long time. "Three and a half weeks after giving birth to Brett, I had so much energy," she says. "My family was amazed at how quickly I regained my strength."

WINNING ACTION

Silence your cravings with healthy substitutions. Most cravings are just too powerful to ignore. Indulging them is fine . . . once in a while. But do it too often, and you could end up gaining weight rather than losing. Instead, try to find nutritious foods that satisfy your hunger without supplying a lot of fat or calories. If you want something crunchy, for example, choose carrot sticks over potato chips. If chocolate is your weakness, opt for fat-free chocolate milk rather than double-fudge ice cream. Save the chips or ice cream as a reward for eating well the rest of the week.

KIDS' PLAYTIME IS MOM'S EXERCISE TIME

Three-year-old Christopher Kautz and his 2-year-old brother, Charlie, are already learning the importance of an active lifestyle. Their mom, Christina, includes them in her workouts whenever she can. For the boys, it's playtime. For Christina, it's an opportunity to bond with her sons while keeping herself slim and shapely.

While pregnant with Christopher, Christina added 45 pounds to her 5-foot-3, 145-pound frame. "By the time I left the maternity ward 3 days after delivery, I had already lost 25," she says. She hoped that the rest of the weight would disappear just as quickly.

To help it along, Christina began exercising as soon as she was able. "We live in Ocean Grove, New Jersey, just two blocks from the ocean," says the 25-year-old mother of two. "I'd walk 2 to 7 miles on the beach, with my son in a backpack. Sometimes I'd walk on the boardwalk, using a jogging stroller."

When she felt ready, Christina gradually trained herself to run. "Each time I went out, I made my turnaround point farther away, increasing my distance a little at a time," she says. "Sometimes I'd take my son along for the ride." She alternated between walking and running, depending on how energetic she felt on any given day.

Her commitment to exercise enabled Christina to return to her prepregnancy weight within 7 months of delivering Christopher. She stayed there until she became pregnant again.

"I gained 37 pounds with Charlie," Christina recalls. "As with Christopher, I lost much of the weight right away, the rest within 4 to 5 months."

Of course, with a toddler and an infant to care for, squeezing in regular workouts required some creativity on Christina's part. She was up to the challenge. "You have to either find time or make time," she explains. "And you have to use it wisely."

For Christina, that meant combining her exercise sessions with her sons' playtime. "My boys have always been 15 to 20 pounds apart, so lifting them helped to strengthen my arms," she says. "They loved being the 'weight' that I would bench-press."

Christina has other ingenious suggestions for exercising with kids. "Doing abdominal crunches with your baby sitting at your feet is a good workout for you and a game of peekaboo for your child," she says. "Pushing a swing works the muscles in your arms and chest quite nicely."

Even though Christina has stayed at her goal weight, she continues to look for fun ways to keep herself and her sons active. "As mothers, we become convinced that we don't have time to take care of ourselves," she says. "I believe that every woman has the opportunity to exercise, no matter how many children she has or how young they are. She just has to look for it."

Christina sees another advantage to getting her sons involved in her fitness routine. "As young as they are, they already seem to know that physical activity is an essential part of every day," she says. "I hope that as a family, we will stay fit and active throughout our lives."

WINNING ACTION

Turn exercise into child's play. *Christina makes a valid point about moms being pressed for time. That's why her idea of combining her workouts with her children's play sessions makes so much sense. Of course, what you do depends on how old your kids are. With an infant or toddler, you can do Christina's overhead lifts and "peekaboo crunches." With older children, you may want to try a game like tag, hide-and-seek, or kickball. You can get other ideas just by watching your kids at play.*

GIVING BIRTH DIDN'T STOP HER FROM GETTING FIT

Through two stints as a mom-to-be, Susannah Devine did all that she could to nurture her growing babies. But her commitment to a healthy lifestyle didn't end once she gave birth. The same eating and exercise habits that supported her pregnancies would ultimately help her shed all but a few pounds of baby fat.

As a certified fitness instructor, Susannah understood the importance of eating well and staying active while she was pregnant. "I had seen so many women with healthy, nonrisk pregnancies stop exercising by their second trimesters," says the 39-year-old Chester, New York, resident. "Staying active is not just natural, it's necessary."

For her part, Susannah kept fit by taking and teaching classes in step aerobics, regular aerobics, and body shaping (which involves strengthening and stretching exercises, plus some yoga movements). She continued her workouts all the way through both of her pregnancies, though she did reduce her level of exertion as her due dates approached. This fitness routine helped her keep a tight rein on her prenatal weight gain. She picked up just 35 pounds with daughter Danielle, who's 13, and 30 pounds with son Devin, who's 9 months.

Once she had her children, Susannah didn't waste time getting back in shape. She was working out just 5 to 6 weeks after each delivery. Of course, she found herself swept up in the same whirlwind of feedings, diaper changes, and naps that threatens to derail many a postpartum weight-loss plan. But she never let it get the best of her.

"My cardinal rule was to ask for help when I needed it," Susannah says. "After my first pregnancy, I had a barter arrangement with another mom. She watched Danielle 2 days a week, and I did the same for her son. After my second pregnancy, I hired the niece of a friend to keep an eye on Devin. She came to the house just twice a week, but that was invaluable to me."

If she needed more time to herself—whether to work out or to do other things—Susannah never hesitated to ask her husband or a relative to watch the kids. "They truly treasured that time with Danielle and Devin," she says. "And they didn't think any less of me because I wanted a couple of extra hours alone."

By opening these "windows" in her schedule, Susannah was able to continue her fitness routine after her pregnancies. The same sense of commitment that had enabled her to control her prenatal weight gain gradually helped her to shed her postpregnancy pounds. "Everything that I had done for my babies I was doing for me," she says. "I was taking care of myself for a change."

Even though 12 years passed between her two pregnancies, Susannah slimmed down faster the second time around (9 months compared with 1½ years). She's holding steady at 124 pounds—slightly above her prepregnancy weight, but appropriate for her 5-foot-6 frame. She's comfortable with her body and her life. To other moms, she offers these words of wisdom: "Enjoy your children and all that they bring to your world. But don't lose sight of yourself."

WINNING ACTION

Maintain the habits of a healthy pregnancy. *One of the advantages of pregnancy is that it can help you change your lifestyle for the better. So once you've had your baby, why not keep a good thing going? After all, you've been eating nutritiously and exercising regularly for 9 months. That's more than enough time for any adjustments that you've made in your lifestyle to become routine.*

FOR HER FIGURE'S SAKE, SHE SWORE OFF FAST FOOD

Cravings for fast food really did a number on Julene Cole's waistline during her second pregnancy. So when she learned that a third child was on the way, the 33-year-old Corona, California, resident didn't trust her willpower to keep her out of the local drive-thrus. What did? Her wallet.

Julene's struggles with her weight didn't really begin until after her second son, Jacob, was born. Her first pregnancy, with son Eddy, went without a hitch. But while carrying Jacob, she developed an almost insatiable appetite for fast food. "I ate a Whopper almost every day!" she recalls. "I'm sure that had a lot to do with my weight gain." She's probably right, considering that each of those burgers supplies 680 calories.

After giving birth to Jacob, Julene was left with a whopping 100 extra pounds on her 5-foot-8½, 155-pound body. She lost 60 rather quickly, but the remaining 40 just wouldn't budge. "I became obsessed with dieting, trying to shed those last 40 pounds," she says. "I tried a lot of unhealthy things, like a green-beans-and-toast diet, with no permanent results."

After 4 years and multiple attempts to slim down—"I lost more self-confidence than weight," she says—Julene finally vented her frustrations to her doctor. He suggested that her birth control method, Depo-Provera injections, might have been preventing her from shedding her baby fat. "Knowing that I wasn't at fault actually made me feel a little better," she says. "I stopped getting the shots, and I started eating nutritiously and walking regularly. Lo and behold, I started losing weight." She was down to 175 pounds when she learned that she was expecting yet again.

This time, Julene resolved not to gain as much weight. She

knew that the trips to the fast-food drive-thru had to stop. "But I couldn't rely on my willpower alone," she says. "The only way I kept myself from eating that stuff was to not take money with me whenever I went somewhere."

Her strategy worked, though Julene admits that living without fast food has been tough on her and her sons Eddy (now age 13) and Jacob (age 5). "The kids definitely miss our burger runs," she says. "If it were up to them, we'd be having fast food every day." As for Julene, she doesn't like cooking all that much, so eating out is a constant temptation. "It's so much easier," she says.

Still, she can't deny that forgoing fast food paid off. She gained 65 pounds over the course of her third pregnancy, but she lost all of that baby fat within a few months of giving birth to her third son, Alex, in May 2000. "Now my goal is to finally lose the leftover pounds from my second pregnancy, with Jacob," she says. "I'd love to get down to between 145 and 155 pounds." By eating right, exercising regularly, and of course, leaving her wallet at home, she stands an excellent chance of achieving lasting weight-loss success.

WINNING ACTION

Find ways to foil fast-food fixes. No one is suggesting that an occasional trip to the nearest drive-thru will cause irreparable damage to your waistline. <u>Occasional</u> is the operative word here. Eating high-fat, high-calorie fast food on a regular basis can run up the scale much higher than is considered healthy, either during or after pregnancy. If the temptation is too great, follow Julene's lead and leave your wallet at home (or at least stash it in the trunk, where it's harder to reach). If the kids insist on going to their favorite burger joint, scan the menu for a *healthier item, such as a grilled chicken sandwich (without mayonnaise or "special sauce") or an entrée salad (with fat-free dressing).*

SHE'S ACTIVELY SETTING A GOOD EXAMPLE FOR HER KIDS

Cheri Spirito couldn't wait to get back in shape after delivering twin sons Justin and Michael in September 1998. She headed back to the gym as soon as she felt able, with her doctor's blessing and her babies in tow. Even though the twins could only watch, she believed that her workout time would do all three of them a world of good.

Cheri hadn't always been so fitness-conscious. She picked up that from her husband, Gene, shortly after they got married. "Both of us had always been careful about our eating habits, but my husband was very active, too," explains the 30-year-old Jeffersonville, Pennsylvania, native. "That convinced me to start working out on a regular basis." She was a trim and toned 5 feet 7, 137 pounds when she became pregnant.

From the start of her pregnancy, Cheri had to limit her activity. Even that didn't prevent her from going into premature labor in her sixth month. "At that point, my doctor ordered me to stay in bed," she recalls. "I couldn't shower, or wash my hair, or put on makeup. I had 'toilet privileges,' but even that could have triggered contractions."

While on bed rest, Cheri gained more than 85 pounds. "My body had gotten so used to being active that when I was knocked off my feet, the weight just piled on," she says. Some of it—about 30

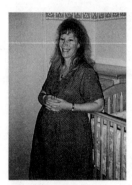
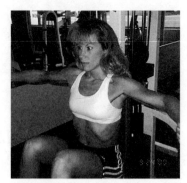

6½ months pregnant   2 years after delivery

pounds—slipped away right after delivery. But the rest didn't budge so easily.

Eager to slim down, Cheri began taking aerobics classes and lifting weights at a local gym. She took Justin and Michael—then about 2 months old—with her, leaving them with the gym's child-care staff while she worked out. "It gave the boys some time away from me, with other children their own age, which I think is important," she says. "It also allowed them to see me being active, which I hope will encourage them to stay fit as they get older."

Within 9 months of starting her workouts, Cheri shed the 55 pounds left behind by her pregnancy. She also earned her certification as an aerobics instructor. "My sister-in-law mentioned that she was getting her certification, and I decided to join her," she says. "I was spending so much time at the gym that I figured, 'Why not get paid to stay in shape?'"

Between teaching step aerobics classes two times a week and continuing her own fitness regimen, Cheri has easily maintained her weight at 137 pounds. "Nobody can believe that I've had twins," she says proudly. "I'm in better shape now than before I got pregnant. Now that my sons are mobile, I don't think they will let me slow down!"

WINNING ACTION

Find time for fitness—for your kids' sake. *Cheri had a wonderfully healthy attitude toward postpartum exercise. Rather than telling herself that she shouldn't spend time away from her babies, as new moms tend to do, she realized that she would help herself and her sons by getting back into her workout regimen. Even at such a young age, children can benefit from exposure to an active lifestyle. They'll grow up to view exercise as a natural, necessary function, just like eating. And they'll emulate your commitment to fitness. So shake off the notion that making time for exercise is selfish. On the contrary, you're doing something wonderful for your kids—and your figure.*

SHE STOPPED GIVING IN TO HER FAMILY'S FOOD WHIMS

Most women would love to have a husband who dabbles in gourmet cooking. Not that Lisa Bowditch is complaining. But between her spouse plying her with rich dishes and her kids begging her for fast food, her chances of ever regaining her prepregnancy figure seemed, well, slim.

Lisa's battle with baby fat began after giving birth to her oldest son, Tyler, in April 1993. Even today, the 34-year-old Uxbridge, Ontario, resident is mortified by photos of her with 60 extra pounds packed on to her petite 5-foot-1, 125-pound body. "I saw my first pregnancy as an excuse to eat junk," she confesses.

When she became pregnant again 2 years later, Lisa was still 20 pounds over her prepregnancy weight. But she had learned her lesson. This time around, she made sure to take care of herself, eating more fruits and vegetables and walking three times a week. "It paid off, because I lost the 35 pounds that I had gained through my pregnancy within 6 weeks of giving birth to my second son, Tanner, in July 1995," she says.

Eager to slim down even more, Lisa signed up for Weight Watchers. "The weekly weigh-ins were a great motivator for me," she says. Within 11 weeks, she lost another 33 pounds. "I was ecstatic with my new figure—and so was my husband," she says. "He had never seen me so slim!"

Lisa maintained her weight for 4 months before she and her husband decided to try for a third child. "Knowing that I was going to be adding pounds anyway, I got careless with my eating habits," she says. "Before I knew it, I was back up to 140."

With two preschool boys to feed, Lisa often found herself pulling into the McDonald's drive-thru for a quick and easy weekday meal. "I'd try not to get anything for myself, but I couldn't resist nibbling on the fries," she says. On weekends, her husband would spend hours in the kitchen preparing tantalizing—and calorie-packed—gourmet entrées that he served with fine wine, freshly baked bread, and a spectacular dessert.

When Lisa became pregnant for a third time in September 1999, she knew that she had to rein in her eating habits. She was not about to repeat the 60-pound weight gain of her first pregnancy. "As much as I appreciate my husband cooking for me, I insisted that he use low-fat recipes whenever possible," she says. "He developed a real knack for ingredient substitution and improvisation."

As for her kids, Lisa continued to treat them to meals from the fast-food drive-thru. But rather than picking at their french fries, she learned to order more healthful menu items for herself, like roasted chicken sandwiches, baked potatoes, and salads.

Lisa found smart ways to accommodate her family's food preferences without losing control of her own eating habits. As a result, she held her prenatal weight gain to just 36 pounds. Six weeks after giving birth to her third son, Troy, in June 2000, she had lost all but 6 of those pounds. "My goal is to slim down to 125, which is what I weighed on my wedding day," she says. "With three sons, I can assume that I have a very active life ahead of me. I want to be able to keep up with them."

W I N N I N G   A C T I O N

Stand guard against the family weight-loss saboteurs. *In trying to please your family's tastebuds, you can easily sabotage your own weight-loss efforts. Instead, look for ways to compromise on your food choices. If your spouse enjoys his meat-and-potatoes meals, make a couple of side dishes to go with them. Then fill your plate with large portions of the veggies and only a small portion of the meat. If your kids want burgers and fries, treat them to lunch at the local fast-food joint. Most of these restaurants now offer menu items that are at least moderately nutritious. The point is, don't just eat something because it's what everyone else wants. Eat what's good for _you_.*

SHE FOUND FITNESS RIGHT OUTSIDE HER FRONT DOOR

While city life isn't for everyone, it suits Melanie Donenfeld just fine. In fact, it helped this 34-year-old mother of two lose a total of 80 postpregnancy pounds.

Melanie and her family—husband Mark and sons Daniel and Matthew—make their home in Manhattan. She walks just about everywhere. "I'm always telling my husband that if we ever move out of the city, I'll probably gain 10 pounds," she says.

Melanie's preference for perambulation paid off once she gave birth to Daniel in December 1995. Over the course of her pregnancy, she added 38 pounds to her 5-foot-6, 120-pound frame. "About half of the extra weight came off within a week," she says. "The rest needed some coaxing to disappear."

Before Daniel's arrival, Melanie had been a full-time public accountant. She decided to go part-time so that she could be with her son. Still, she didn't want to become sedentary, lest those postpartum pounds become permanent. So she went walking at every opportunity—whether to run errands, to visit friends, or just to get some air. "I would push Daniel in his stroller," she says. "We probably covered between 1 and 3 miles a day."

Over the course of 2½ months, Melanie walked off every last ounce of baby fat. But nearly 2 years later, when she became pregnant with Matthew, she wondered whether she could repeat her weight-loss success. "I was a few years older, and I had two children to care for rather than one," she says.

After delivering Matthew in May 1998, Melanie found herself padded with 42 extra pounds—a few more than from her first pregnancy. Eager to slim down, she signed up for a Strollercise class, in which participants run with their babies in strollers, stopping at designated points to do exercises. "It seemed like a good idea, since I had two children still in strollers," she says. "But the structure of the class didn't appeal to me."

Melanie decided to stick with ordinary walking, which had proven its weight-loss merits after her first pregnancy. She trekked all over Manhattan, this time with both boys in tow. She lost all but one of her postpregnancy pounds in about 6 months. "It took longer than the first time around, most likely because I was older and because I ate a lot more junk food while carrying Matthew," she says.

Even though she's no longer worried about baby fat, Melanie continues to make tracks around Manhattan. "I love walking," she says. "Now when I need to go somewhere, I think twice about getting in a bus or cab. I'd really rather walk."

WINNING ACTION

Explore the exercise opportunities in your hometown.
Even if you don't live in a major metropolitan area, as Melanie does, you can probably find lots of interesting ways to spice up your fitness routine right in your own backyard. Perhaps your community has established self-guided walking tours of its gardens or historic districts. Maybe the local park has a fitness course (which features exercise "stations" spread out over the length of the course), mountain-biking trails, or an ice-skating rink. Your community's parks and recreation department, or its tourist information office, can fill you in on the details.

DAUGHTER'S DAIRY DILEMMA SAVED THIS MOM'S FIGURE

To look at Sara Straub now, you'd never guess that the 28-year-old mother of four from River Heights, Utah, once weighed close to 200 pounds. She might still be heavy, were it not for the fact that she had to give up dairy products in order to continue breastfeeding her youngest daughter. That single dietary change enabled Sara to shed 61 pounds of baby fat.

When she became pregnant for the first time—with her son Ian, now 9—Sara was slightly underweight for her build: 5 feet 6 and 117 pounds. Her doctor told her that she'd need to gain more weight than normally recommended in order to support her growing baby. She put on 60 pounds before giving birth to Ian, then worked off all but 12 of those pounds within 5 months by riding her stationary bicycle and walking.

Through her next three pregnancies—with 6-year-old Samantha, 4-year-old Caleb, and 1-year-old Isobel—Sara watched her weight continue to creep upward. "Actually, the roughest spot was between my pregnancies with Caleb and Isobel," she says. "We moved into a new home, and I guess I got a little lazy. I ended up gaining 20 pounds, plus another 30 with Isobel."

Once considered too thin, this young mom could hardly believe that she had reached 186 pounds. But that's what the scale read when she weighed in a few days after delivering Isobel. "Seeing that number convinced me that I had to make changes," Sara recalls. "I had never, ever imagined myself becoming overweight."

But she had little time to strategize her weight-loss plan. Shortly after she started breastfeeding Isobel, she discovered that her baby girl was lactose intolerant. That meant Sara had to forgo all dairy products for as long as she was nursing. "Dairy was a big part of my diet.

I loved my milk, butter, and cheese," she says. "Giving them up wasn't easy, but I had no choice. They made my daughter scream in agony."

But little Isobel wasn't the only one to benefit from her mom's dietary change. Sara discovered that once she cut out those high-fat, high-calorie dairy products, the excess weight left behind by her pregnancies began to melt away. "That encouraged me to do more to slim down," she says. "I felt capable of succeeding, which was an incredible motivator."

Sara started swimming every morning and lifting weights at home three times a week. To ensure that she got enough calcium, she ate nondairy foods rich in the mineral, like broccoli and spinach, and drank soy milk. She also took calcium supplements.

Over the course of 6 months, Sara lost 61 pounds. At 125, she's a few pounds heavier than before her pregnancies, but happy with her weight. "I feel great!" she exclaims. "I have so much more energy now that I'm eating better."

WINNING ACTION

Seek out alternative sources of calcium. *Dairy products are outstanding sources of calcium, a mineral that's important for all women, especially nursing moms. Unfortunately, it's often accompanied by unhealthy doses of fat and calories—not what you want when you're trying to slim down. You can get calcium from nondairy foods, like oysters, cauliflower, and calcium-enriched fruit juices. You can also opt for low-fat and fat-free dairy products, including cheeses, yogurt, and milk. Either way, you'll shore up your calcium supply while supporting your weight-loss goals.*

SHE'S ALL JAZZED UP
TO SLIM DOWN

Laura Tant is no fan of exercise. But that doesn't stop her from working out twice a week. As long as she's listening to music, she gets into the moves. She's counting on them to whittle away the pounds from her third pregnancy.

Before she started having kids, Laura never worried about her weight. "I wasn't all that active, and I certainly didn't diet," says the 23-year-old Fayetteville, Georgia, resident. "To this day, Oreos are my favorite food."

Whether because of good genes or a speedy metabolism, Laura maintained her 5-foot-8 figure at 145 pounds. Then she got married and gave birth to son Bear, who's now 5, and daughter Glynis, who's 3. Suddenly, her body seemed to be playing by a new set of rules. It just clung to the baby fat, especially after Glynis was born.

With her scale stuck at 160, Laura's self-esteem plummeted, only to suffer a greater blow when Laura and her husband decided to divorce. "I felt so alone, yet I had gained so much weight that I couldn't imagine anyone going out with me," she says.

Laura wanted to reclaim her prepregnancy figure in the worst way. She knew that regular exercise would help melt away the pounds. But it just seemed so boring.

Then a friend suggested that Laura try Jazzercise, a form of aerobic exercise that's choreographed and set to music. Somewhat reluctantly, Laura attended her first class about 6 months after Glynis was born. To her surprise, she really enjoyed it. "The music made such a difference," she says. "And the other women in the class were so friendly and supportive. They encouraged me to stick with it."

Laura took their advice, attending Jazzercise classes at least twice a week. Within a matter of months, she was back to her prepregnancy weight of 145.

Since then, Laura has remarried and given birth to another daughter, Corynn, who's now 15 months. The pregnancy pushed Laura's weight back up to 155, but she's not panicking about those extra pounds. She's still taking the Jazzercise classes, confident that she'll slim down just like before.

According to this former fitness-phobe, music is what keeps her going back to the gym. "I don't feel bored, which turned me off to most forms of exercise," she says. "I'm not crazy about Ricky Martin, but even his songs are great for working out!"

WINNING ACTION

Set your moves to music. *A 30-minute workout will go so much faster when it's set to your favorite tunes. In fact, depending on your activity of choice, music can help you maintain a steady, heart-pumping pace. You can buy prerecorded aerobics and walking tapes with a set tempo. Or you can make a tape from your own audio collection. Just be careful with the pace: You want to go fast, but not so fast that you can't talk without gasping for air.*

FOR THIS MOM, FLATTERY IS THE SINCEREST FORM OF INSPIRATION

Every woman likes to be told how fabulous she looks. Sarah Jane Mewshaw is no different. In fact, she credits a few well-timed compliments with rescuing her weight-loss efforts and renewing her commitment to a healthy lifestyle.

At 5 feet 9 and 145 pounds, Sarah weighs now what she did in

1990, before she began having children. But maintaining her trim figure hasn't been easy. Her struggles began while she was pregnant with her son, Andrew, who's now 10. "I didn't watch what I ate, and I didn't exercise," recalls Sarah, a 34-year-old resident of Naples, Florida. "I paid for that eventually."

She gained 40 pounds through her first pregnancy, but lost only 18. She weighed 167 pounds when she became pregnant with her daughter, Caitlin, who's now 6. "I certainly didn't want to get any heavier, so I took better care of myself," she says. "I paid more attention to my food choices, and I took up walking to get fit."

Sarah succeeded in controlling her weight gain the second time around, putting on just 15 pounds. Not only that, just months after delivering her daughter, she was down to 140 pounds. After 2 years, she leveled out at 145, where she has held steady ever since.

Sarah knows that abandoning her healthy lifestyle would have a negative effect on her waistline. For this reason, she has stepped up her fitness routine, engaging in high-intensity running and walking as much as she can. She has also made some improvements in her dietary habits, cutting back on fried foods, snacking on fruits instead of junk food, and drinking more water.

Even though she has managed to keep off the extra pounds, Sarah sometimes feels that she's fighting an uphill battle against Mother Nature. Invariably, those are the moments when she runs into someone whom she hasn't seen in a while, and she's told how marvelous she looks. "It's uncanny, really," she muses. "Just when I might be entertaining the notion of abandoning my healthy habits, someone comes along to remind me why I shouldn't."

Sarah still wants to lose a few more pounds, so that she's even slimmer than before she had her children. She knows that she'll need to be extravigilant about eating healthfully and exercising regularly. She's counting on the kind words of old acquaintances to help her succeed. "Getting compliments from people whom I haven't seen in ages really energizes me," she says. "It got me this far. I'm sure it can take me even further."

W I N N I N G   A C T I O N

Use compliments as the spark to fire up your motivation. *Losing those postpregnancy pounds takes time and effort. As a result, you may not see the changes in your body, because they are gradual. But the people around you can. So when someone pays you a compliment about your figure, accept it as an acknowledgment of what you've accomplished. Use it as inspiration to continue pursuing your weight-loss goals. You might even turn it into an affirmation that you can repeat to yourself whenever you need to lift your spirits: "I am getting thinner and looking better every day" or a similar phrase that motivates you.*

LEAD THIS MOM TO WATER— AND SHE'LL LOSE WEIGHT

Over the course of three pregnancies, Cynthia Fuller gained and lost a total of 103 pounds. The 35-year-old paralegal from Chiefland, Florida, found the secret of weight-loss success in a bottle—a water bottle.

A former model, Cynthia was accustomed to carrying about 140 pounds on her 6-foot frame. So when her weight climbed to

193 after her third pregnancy, she couldn't wait to get rid of the baby fat. "The extra pounds really bothered me," she says. "I felt very unhealthy and not all that attractive."

With a full-time job and three children to look after—Madison, who's now 8; Dylan, 6; and Nicholas, 4—Cynthia didn't have much time for exercise. "Coaching soccer, volleyball, and T-ball kept me active," she says. It also tipped her off to the incredible pound-paring powers of water.

During the seasons when she's coaching, Cynthia drinks between 10 and 12 bottles of water (16.9 ounces each) a day. She figured that if she could stretch her water habit year-round, she'd be able to drop those unwanted postpregnancy pounds *pronto*.

Cynthia aimed to drink at least six bottles of water a day. Sure enough, as her intake increased, the pounds melted away. Within the year after her youngest son, Nicholas, was born, her weight dropped to 150. It has stayed there ever since. "For someone of my height, 145 to 150 is ideal," she explains.

For Cynthia, drinking water has become a ritual that not only enables her to maintain her weight but also enhances her health in other ways. "I need to take care of myself, so I can always take care of my kids," she says. "That means more to me than anything."

WINNING ACTION

Drink at least eight 8-ounce glasses of water a day. *Although it gets little respect, water has so many health benefits that your kitchen tap could be called a fountain of youth. Drinking lots of water supports weight loss by preventing dehydration, which disrupts your body's metabolism. In one study, conducted at the University of Utah in Salt Lake City, researchers found that volunteers* *who were already dehydrated from using diuretics burned fewer calories <u>after</u> a period of stationary cycling than before the exercise session started.*

In addition, drinking water before a meal makes you feel full, so you eat less. It does other good things for you as well: It keeps you alert, makes your skin glow, and reduces your risk of many diseases.

You don't have to drink as much water as Cynthia to experience its positive effects. Just eight 8-ounce glasses a day is enough. If you prefer, you can buy a single 64-ounce bottle, then keep it with you and take frequent sips from it throughout the day.

PAPER ROUTE DELIVERS THE BODY SHE WANTS

Many moms-to-be worry about gaining weight during pregnancy. Misty Weaver-Ostinato actually looked forward to it. At 5 feet 7 and 95 pounds, Misty was exceptionally thin, as she had been for most of her life. When she became pregnant in April 1998, she saw her opportunity to add a few pounds.

Misty gained 35 pounds before giving birth to daughter Summer in November 1998. She quickly lost 20 of them—"mostly baby weight and amniotic fluid," says the 24-year-old Dumfries, Virginia, native. Summer was just 4 months old when her mom became pregnant again. "I went into premature labor three times," Misty recalls. "I was on complete bed rest for 3 months, and I delivered 2 months early."

She gained 40 pounds before giving birth to son Tyler in October 1999. Just as after her first pregnancy, she quickly shed much of the weight, dropping down to 125.

While happy with the extra pounds, Misty realized that she had gotten out of shape, especially after being on extended bed rest. She had been active throughout high school and college, and she wanted to start exercising again. She found an unusual way to do it.

"A friend of mine owns a newspaper distributorship, and he was going on vacation," Misty says. "I offered to help him out by taking one of his paper routes. I'd do my deliveries early in the morning, while my children were sleeping and my husband was at home to take care of them."

The job started when Tyler was about 6 months old, and it lasted just 2 weeks. But that was long enough for Misty to lose another 10 pounds—"mostly from sweating," she says. "It was 85° outside, and I was bagging newspapers in the back of a semi with no air-conditioning!"

Misty has held steady at 115, which is 20 pounds above her prepregnancy weight. She's extremely happy with her new figure, which she keeps in shape by walking and running after her two toddlers. She learned so much through her two pregnancies that she has even started her own Web site, MomsHelpMoms.com, to provide information to stay-at-home and working moms. "I put it together for my family and friends, but it has grown tremendously," she says. "Now I employ three people, and I'm having so much fun!"

WINNING ACTION

Walk like you're on a mission. *Walking is a wonderful activity for losing postpregnancy pounds. It's low-impact, so it's gentle to your body. And when done at a moderate* *to brisk pace, it can burn plenty of calories. If you're not content to just look at the scenery, think of ways to add purpose to your workouts. Do your errands on foot. Trim your lawn with a push mower. Take your dog for a walk—or if you don't have one, volunteer as a dog-walker at your local animal shelter. You can even follow Misty's lead and get a paper route. You'll get your exercise—and a little extra cash to boot!*

THIS MOM GAVE UP SWEETS FOR CAKE

Cake plays an important role in Jody Eastridge's life. No, it's not quite what you think. In fact, it's much better than any pastry chef's creation. CAKE is Jody's acronym for her children—quadruplets Chad, Amanda, Katie, and Emily, who were born in April 1998.

For Jody and her husband, Mike, the quads' arrival was the joyous culmination of 10 years spent trying to conceive. "We finally opted for in vitro fertilization," says Jody, 32, who lives with her family in Amana, Iowa. "We were in that 1 percent of people for whom all of the eggs take!"

That happened in September 1997. By December, Jody was on complete bed rest, which severely restricted her physical activity. At 5 feet 8 and 235 pounds, she already had a weight problem when she became pregnant. Now a lack of exercise threatened to pile on even more pounds.

Sure enough, by the quads' delivery date, Jody reached her highest weight of 270 pounds. But to her pleasant surprise, 50 of those pounds disappeared within 2 days. She had lost all of the baby fat, and then some. "Actually, I didn't even gain as much as I had expected, considering that from week 13 on, I went out only on Fridays for a doctor's appointment," she says.

Much to Jody's chagrin, however, the weight she had so easily lost right after delivery slowly began to return. "I wasn't getting much exercise, and on top of that, I was polishing off whatever the kids left on their plates," she recalls. Within 2 years, she was back to 270 pounds.

Realizing that she had regained all of her prenatal weight, Jody snapped into action. "I had to get fit and healthy for my kids," she says. "I didn't want them to be embarrassed by their mom as they got older."

Jody's first step was to stop bringing candy and ice cream into her house. "If it's not here, I won't want it!" she says. Next, she banned fried foods, as well as late-night suppers. "I make sure that we eat before 6 o'clock," she says.

Eventually, Jody joined Inches-A-Weigh, a health club and support group exclusively for women who want to slim down. "I have to drive 40 minutes to get there, but I really like it," she says. "There's a nutritionist on-site, as well as 10 figure-shaping machines for a low-impact, low-exertion workout." She goes to exercise for up to an hour twice a week.

Jody gets a lot of support from her husband, too. "Mike hurries home to watch the kids so that I can go work out," she says. "And since I've been eating healthier, he is, too."

Since joining Inches-A-Weigh, Jody has lost 24 pounds. Perhaps more important, she has come to understand that the key to lasting weight-loss success lies in permanent lifestyle modification. "Dieting alone won't do it," she says. "It requires a total turnaround of thoughts and behaviors." This retraining takes some time and effort, but it's worthwhile in the long run, in terms of your weight and your overall health.

"You can teach your tastebuds that salads are better than candy," Jody affirms. For her, of course, nothing is as good as CAKE.

WINNING ACTION

Recognize that permanent weight loss requires permanent change. *Many people diet until they reach their goal weights, then revert to their old, unhealthy habits. Invariably, their pounds return—often with accomplices. If you want that baby fat gone for good, you must make lasting, positive changes in your eating and exercise habits. But don't make them all at once. You're better off tackling them one by one, in baby steps. For example, if you want to cut butter or margarine from your meals, start by substituting fruit spread on your toast at breakfast. If you want to walk for 30 minutes every day, start with 5. This approach makes the changes manageable and your progress measurable.*

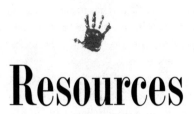

Resources

A STRENGTH-TRAINING ROUTINE FOR NEW MOMS

The road to postpartum fitness has to start somewhere. Why not in your own home? Even in the busy weeks immediately following your pregnancy, daily practice of a few basic exercises can help speed up the recovery process.

In general, women are ready to resume a regular fitness routine about 6 weeks after giving birth. The time frame can vary, based on the circumstances surrounding delivery. If you had a cesarean section or episiotomy, for example, you may need longer to recuperate. That's why you should check with your doctor before you start working out.

The exercises presented below are ideal for new moms. They can be done on a daily basis (depending on how you feel), perhaps while baby naps or plays close by. They're recommended by Shari Brasner, M.D., a board-certified obstetrician and gynecologist and faculty member at Mount Sinai School of Medicine in New York City, and Craig Cisar, Ph.D., professor of exercise physiology in the department of human performance at San Jose State University in California.

Abdominal crunches. Lie on your back with your knees bent. Fold your arms across your chest so that your fingertips touch your shoulders. Squeeze your abdominal muscles so that the small of your back is flat against the floor. Inhale as you raise your head slightly and look at your lower abdomen. Exhale as you hold this position for 3 seconds, then return to the starting position. Repeat 10 times.

Each week, increase the number of crunches you perform and the number of seconds you hold them by one. For example, in the second week, do 11 crunches, holding each for 4 seconds.

Pelvic tilts. Lie on your back with your knees bent. Inhale as you raise your buttocks and contract your stomach muscles. Hold for 5 seconds, then slowly lower your buttocks, feeling each vertebra make contact with the floor. Repeat 10 times, increasing by two per week.

Inner thigh lifts. Lie on your right side, supporting yourself on your right elbow. Position your left hand in front of your body. Bend your left knee and position your left foot behind your right knee. Raise your right leg as high as you can, keeping your toes pointed. Slowly lower your leg. Repeat the motion, this time flexing your foot forward. Repeat the exercise 10 times, alternating between pointed toes and flexed foot (5 times each). Then switch sides. Increase the number of repetitions by two per week.

Modified pushups. Lie on your stomach with your hands at least shoulder-width apart. Inhale as you raise your upper body, keeping your knees on the floor. Exhale as you lower your body, but don't go all the way to the floor. Repeat 10 times to start, increasing the number of repetitions by two each week.

Arm lifts. Lie on your stomach with your arms stretched out in front of you. Inhale as you raise your head and lift both arms, stretching up and out. Exhale as you hold for 5 seconds, then slowly return to the starting position. Repeat 10 times, increasing the number of repetitions by two per week.

Fire hydrants. Kneel with your hands, forearms, and elbows on the floor. Inhale, and keeping your knee bent, raise your right leg out to the side so that your thigh is parallel with the floor. Exhale as you return to the starting position. Repeat 10 times, then switch sides. Increase the number of repetitions by two per week.

Triceps chair pushups. Sit on the edge of a sturdy chair with your hands grasping the edge of the seat. Your hands should be about shoulder-width apart, and your knees bent at about 90 degrees to stabilize your position. Inhale as you lower your body as far as you can, but don't sit down. Exhale as you use your arms to push yourself back onto the chair. Be sure your legs are far enough away that you're working arm and shoulder muscles. Repeat 10 times, increasing the number of repetitions by two per week.

Squats. Stand in front of a chair as if you're about to sit down on it, with your hands on your hips or hanging alongside your body, and your feet shoulder-width apart. Inhale as you lower your body, but stop a few inches above the seat. Keep your back and lower legs as straight as possible, using only your buttock and thigh muscles to perform the movement. Exhale as you return to a standing position. Repeat 10 times, increasing the number of repetitions by two per week.

Toe touches. Sit on the floor with your legs stretched out in front of you. Exhale as you reach for your ankles or calves, bending your torso forward and leaning over your thighs. Hold for 10 to 15 seconds, then inhale as you return to an upright position. Repeat three times. Work up to 20 to 30 seconds per stretch and five repetitions.

INDEX

Underscored page references indicate tables,
boxed text, and Winning Action sidebars.

A

B

C

BRADFORD WG LIBRARY
100 HOLLAND COURT, BOX 130
BRADFORD, ONT. L3Z 2A7